Mindfulness for Life

Mindfulness for Life

A Six-Week Guide to Inner Peace

Oli Doyle

Copyright © Oli Doyle 2016

The right of Oli Doyle to be identified as
the author of this work has been asserted in accordance with the
Copyright, Designs and Patents Act 1988.

This edition first published in Great Britain in 2016 by
Orion
an imprint of the Orion Publishing Group Ltd
Carmelite House, 50 Victoria Embankment,
London, EC4Y 0DZ
An Hachette UK Company

1 3 5 7 9 10 8 6 4 2

A CIP catalogue record for this book is available
from the British Library.

Paperback ISBN: 978 1 4091 6066 3

Printed in Great Britain by
CPI Group (UK) Ltd, Croydon, CR0 4YY

The Orion Publishing Group's policy is to use papers that are natural,
renewable and recyclable and made from wood grown in sustainable forests.
The logging and manufacturing processes are expected to conform to the
environmental regulations of the country of origin.

For Ren, Liam and Freya,
my most important teachers

Contents

Introduction

The thing about life is that people seem to suffer, but we don't need to. We can be happy, peaceful and content right now, if we only change a couple of simple things. The normal human approach to this conundrum is laughable when you pull it apart. Humans are unhappy because we spend our time and energy thinking about things that don't exist – the past and the future. Add to this our habit of arguing with life, believing it to be wrong and thinking about why it should be different and you have a potent combination, tailor-made for a life of suffering. Thinking about the past leads to anger, regret, sadness and grief. Thinking about the future causes stress, anxiety, worry and fear. And neither of them exists. The irony of this situation is that life, which is happening now, is filled with peace, quiet and contentment, if only you know where to look, and that brings us to those simple changes that can make a big difference.

Personally, I learnt this lesson the hard way when, at the age of 22, I tried to learn the secrets of meditation from books.

Those books were amazing, written by the likes of the Dalai Lama, but I struggled for years to apply their lessons and techniques because I did not understand the cultural perspective from which they were written. And so I kept searching. I looked outside of myself from teacher to teacher and from technique to technique until one day I discovered that all of meditation, or mindfulness, or whatever you prefer to call it, is about looking within.

As I played with this discovery and my experience of peace and happiness continued to deepen, I decided to write a book. That book, *Mindfulness Plain and Simple*, was an attempt to demystify the simple science of mindful happiness, and to translate the words of the mystics into simple, everyday Western language. It was published back in 2010, and in the years since, my understanding of the processes of mindfulness has deepened. I have reduced that process down to four core skills that complement each other and overlap, but that are a useful way to put mindfulness into practice quickly and easily. Having done this work, I realised that simplifying the practice so deeply could change lives, and that if I could write a book that was both informative and practical, your mindfulness might deepen, even as you read. And so, *Mindfulness for Life* was born.

Mindfulness for Life is designed to maximise your insights and deepen your practice, while making mindfulness skills easier to incorporate into your day. The book is divided into six weeks. The first four look at the following skills:

- instantaneous focus
- allowfulness
- noticing space
- living as awareness.

The final two weeks look at the two most important processes you will go through as your practice deepens:

- dropping obstacles
- waking up from compulsive thinking.

Each week is made up of seven entries – one for each day – that explore seven core themes:

- self-esteem
- dealing with emotions
- mindful relationships
- mindfulness at work
- mindful creativity
- mindfulness and health
- mindfulness for life.

In writing this book I set out to give you an understanding of these skills as well as the opportunity to practise them as you read.

As you will discover within the pages of this book, happiness is as simple as turning your attention to Now and becoming focused on our inner world, although I am aware that those words may not mean much to you ... yet. The purpose of this book is to explain the traps and snares keeping you stuck and, more importantly, to show you the path of freedom. By the end you will have developed a new set of skills that you can hone and refine on your own, and you will have the ability to live in the present moment, to deal with the challenges of life and to develop truly loving relationships with other people.

The method used here is designed to be practical, applicable to daily life and manageable even on a busy day. This is more than a book, it is a mindfulness course that will fit in your backpack.

As you read, don't be constrained by the format, but allow yourself to explore in the way that feels right for you. You might wish to read through the book over six weeks, covering a section each day, or you may want to read sections at random as it occurs to you to do so. Trust that however you approach this work, you will benefit from the practices and new learnings. The weeks do not have to be read sequentially and there is no hierarchy to them, so random or structured will work fine, as long as you put the time into the practices themselves.

Practice need not be arduous or lengthy. Even 10 to 20 minutes each day can make a major difference in your life. Also, the exercises are designed to be as easy to integrate into everyday life as possible.

As you take this journey, remember that getting lost in thought is normal and has been the way for humans for thousands of years. So if you find yourself daydreaming, scheming and thinking, don't fret; this is what almost all humans do, it's just that relatively few are aware that it is happening. As that awareness grows in you, thinking will begin to subside quite naturally.

And finally, remember that the process that is happening through you – humans waking up out of thought – is a significant shift in this world. As you become free of suffering, this freedom will flow on into the world and the people around you. Thank you so much for joining me on this journey, and for bringing a little more peace into this world.

To assist you in your learning, a set of free resources that accompany the course are available at www.olidoyle.com/MFL.

WEEK 1

Learning to Focus

The Most Important Lesson

Everybody knows that everything happens Now – that there is no other moment in time – and that the past and the future are really just thoughts, or memories, or imaginings. We all get that on a conceptual level, but most people don't understand it. Most people don't live it. And that is why human beings are lost; why we are stressed, unhappy and frustrated; and why we live our lives unaware of the power, the peace and the happiness that is within us all the time.

In this book, we will be taking a six-week journey of peace, starting with some basic principles. We'll begin by learning how to shift our attention into this moment. Hundreds (or thousands) of books have been written on the subject, and though we might all know conceptually that living in the present is a good idea, becoming truly present, truly aware, is not an easy thing to do. We will look at the reasons for this in some detail, but more importantly, in this first week, I will give you the tools you need to bring your attention into the present moment. This is the most basic and necessary lesson, and once you have learnt it, all the subsequent skills will be easy to master. I will also show you how to return to Now when you get lost in another thought, which is normal and inevitable.

First, let's examine some of the roadblocks you are likely to encounter along the way. My hope is that by knowing about these in advance, you'll be able to recognise them as a normal part of the process, and not something personally wrong with you or your mindfulness practice. I hope that when you encounter these challenges, you will continue with a small smile rather than giving up or thinking you can't do it. For it is through this continued practice, day after day, that you will begin to see peace and happiness creeping softly into your life.

The Mind's Inability to be Present

The first thing you will notice – even if you have been doing this for years – is that the mind resists any attempt to be present. Each time you make an effort to shift your attention into the present moment, there is a pull back in the other direction. That pull comes from thought. And each thought that arises is focused, quite naturally, not on the present moment but on the past and the future. This is because the mind is essentially drawn to the analytical process. It continually analyses events, trying to make sense of them, looking for patterns, and attempting to use the past to predict the future.

Realising Freedom is Natural

As you go through this book, you will use the experience of really living to open up the door to your true self, which is where freedom will come from – where real freedom is right now. That freedom is our natural state, but we block it with our insistent need to keep thinking and thinking and planning and scheming. But that's OK; that's where we are right now. For years you have been conditioned to listen to your thoughts and to listen to other people's thoughts, opinions and beliefs – even to value those thoughts more than your own experience.

We're so used to listening to our thoughts, we're so obsessed with thoughts, and we're so completely lost in thought as a species (thanks partly to all those years of conditioning) that it is going to take some effort to keep coming back to the present moment. But all you have to do is keep noticing. As soon as you notice you are lost, just come back. Because as soon as you notice you're lost, you're not lost any more. In the moment of noticing, you are awake. Even if you drift back to sleep very quickly, you are awake in that instant. And being awake means that you are present as the observer of thought instead of being completely caught up in it. As you move through this course, don't worry about the times when you fall asleep – just continue to wake up, again and again.

The Inevitability of Getting Lost

As you begin this journey of exploration, I want you to keep in mind that you will get lost again and again and again. I also want you to keep in mind, and in your heart, that your mind doesn't know how your practice is going. Your mind is just commenting and analysing and judging, and while you're lost in that, you're not practising. And when you are practising, your mind isn't in control any more, so your mind can't know what your practice is like. It will want to comment on your practice, but its comments won't be accurate, because it lives in a different world.

The other thing I want you to remember during this week is to watch out for goals. You don't need to try to get rid of them or to tell yourself, 'I'm spiritual; I have no goals,' because that's a goal too. All you need to do is notice when goals are arising, which is basically every time you notice thoughts about the future: what your practice is going to be like or what your life is going to be like when you are calm and peaceful and achieve a Zen state. When you notice those types of thoughts, just come back to your practice today, Now. Come back to the practice again and again. Don't worry about the content of your thoughts. Just become the observer of them; just watch them.

Getting Started

The first tool you will use on this path of mindfulness and self-discovery is what I call instantaneous focus. This means bringing your attention so sharply into this moment that there is no room for anything else – any thought – to take over. Of course, thoughts can still arise (and they will) and that's fine. We're not trying to get rid of thought or to block it. We're not trying to have a quiet mind. We just want to be primarily focused on our object of awareness, which in this practice will be the breath. With instantaneous focus, you are so sharply aware – so alive in this moment – that everything else fades into to the background.

As you become more focused on this instant, you will learn to step out of the story of Me, to step off the conveyor belt and out of the factory altogether. You will learn how to bring your focus into this instant so sharply, so intently, that you completely drop all thinking. You are going to shift from thinking about life to experiencing life. I am going to give you the tools to make that shift through a powerful exercise that will be your daily practice for this week. You can only experience life if your attention is tightly honed in on this moment. And I want you to remember and keep coming back to this: you are not trying to become peaceful; you are just shifting from thinking to experience.

Of course, the story of Me will still go on. Thoughts will still come and go. Millions of things are happening inside and outside of us – coming, going and disappearing – but the primary focal point of your attention and all your awareness will be this one breath, this one instant. (As you get started, you can also head to www.olidoyle.com/MFL and find the exercises that accompany Week 1.)

Day 1: Just You, Just Now

Beyond My Self

To start this plan, I want to turn the idea of self-esteem on its head as we practise the art of not having a self in the first place. This sounds very Zen and esoteric, but in fact it is a simple, practical skill, and here is the key: the self that feels good or bad about itself is no more than a story in your head.

In this instant, no self exists.

Consider this for a moment. Recall every phrase you use to describe yourself and notice how they all come from the past. Everything you can say about your self is a story from before. I could say 'I am a man sitting typing at a computer' and that would be true right now, but that's not a statement about self-esteem, which arises because of the judgements we make about ourselves. If I say, 'I am a very good author,' I am describing a belief about myself based on the past, and this is where the trouble starts!

As soon as we rely on stories to tell us about ourselves, we are in serious trouble on two fronts. Firstly, the mind is rarely positive, and is highly likely to focus on what you haven't done well in the past, which is why most people have problems with their self-esteem. Secondly, while you are busy thinking about what kind of person you are, you're missing out on the present moment, also known as 'life'! In our efforts to please the judging voice in the head, we sacrifice our very own precious life. What a terrible bargain!

The Story of Me

From the belief of creating stories, we each create the story of Me. This story is really just a bundle of thoughts, or beliefs, or experiences that you turn into your sense of self. The answer to 'Who am I?' might include your name, your physical appearance, your mental characteristics, your skills, the things you've done well, the things you haven't, and on and on. By bundling all these together, you create the picture you call Me. However, it's not really the full picture, because it's impossible for the mind to capture everything you've done, everything you've experienced, every skill and perceived flaw. We all just pick a few and bundle them together to form our picture of ourselves.

But what if you just take life an instant at a time? What then? Try it today; any time thoughts arise about what kind of person you are and what sort of job you are doing, shift your focus to the activity you are engaged in this instant. Make the activity itself primary and the story of what it means secondary (the opposite of the usual human way) and see what happens.

Activity: Just This

Choose a simple activity that you do every day, like washing the dishes, brushing your teeth or walking the dog. Spend 5–20 minutes doing that activity for its own sake, with no concern for what it may lead to, or what it says about you. For example, if you walk the dog, simply walk with careful attention, experiencing one step at a time. Forget about the last step, the next step, or how much weight you can lose by walking every day. Just walk. Feel your feet on the ground. Feel each breath in your chest. Stop being a story of Me and just be.

Once you get comfortable with this practice, extend it to other areas in your life. What happens when the activity itself, the process, becomes more important than the outcome? And what happens to the story of me in that moment of just this step, just this breath?

The Obsession with Time

We've seen that the mind is an analytical process, concerned only with the past and future, and particularly, with
what's wrong. It looks for problems and sees fixing them
as its job. It tries to figure out how to keep the problems
from occurring again, or how to get a different result in the
future, so that we can be happy. These are good intentions
– there is nothing wrong with the mind – but you may have
found (and perhaps that is why you picked up this book)
that living lost in thought isn't much fun; living your life
thinking about the past and the future is stressful most of
the time. Sometimes it may be pleasant, but even then it's
not as fulfilling – not anywhere close to as fulfilling – as
spending a moment totally immersed in the Now, in this
present moment. That shift to Now is an instant relief, and
it can be yours with a simple change in focus – from thinking to experiencing life as it is.

When the mind views something about you as the problem, the stress and pain caused by this process is magnified,
as is the relief you will experience when you step out of the
illusion of time and into your true, instantaneous self.

Because of the mind's obsession with the past and future, it
views time as a conveyor belt that runs from the past through
the present to the future. You can look back and know exactly
what came before, and you can look forward and see what
might come next, which gives time the appearance of linear
continuity. When you believe thought, the past seems quite
real, as does the future, but when you trust your actual experience, there is only ever this Now. And as you notice that only
this instant is actually real, the burden of that time-based self

will begin to dissolve. This is the first benefit of a mindful life. No self, no problems.

Day 2: Instantaneous Relationships

The Crowded Room

Bringing instantaneous focus to relationships is incredibly helpful because it takes us out of the history of the relationship. Every relationship has its own history, its own story, and every relationship carries that baggage. As soon as you interact with someone – whether it's the person you've been living with for ten years, or a friend, or someone you've known all your life, like a parent or sibling – you are looking at the person through the mind, and all that history comes to the interaction with you.

Metaphorically speaking, your mind is a crowded room full of voices from the past, all jostling for attention. It's hard to give anyone your full attention because the past keeps coming in and trying to tell you what's important, what to notice and what to ignore.

This often results in interactions that keep following similar patterns – not because we haven't changed as people, but because we are stuck in the same thoughts when we are with the same people. Often it is the story that stays the same, not the people. When you learn to sharpen your attention down to this moment, you can focus just on the time you are spending with the person Now. You can really notice the person's facial expressions today, the way the person is talking today – you can really listen. And in that listening, the relationship changes.

Thoughts are fearful creatures, and they simultaneously desire and fear other people – desiring their approval, love or appreciation; fearful of their rejection, or of being hurt in some way. Whenever two thought-identified humans interact, there is a pattern of desire and fear underneath the interaction. The level of fear depends on the past experiences on which the thoughts are based, so someone who has suffered abuse and humiliation in past relationships is likely to have thought patterns that reflect this, while someone who has had relatively healthy relationships may have lighter thought patterns. But while the severity may differ, if you are lost in thought, the pattern will be there, and it will pollute every relationship eventually. The pollution comes because, when I am lost in this pattern, I am focused on what I can get from the relationship, rather than being focused on you.

When you speak, I am thinking about what it means for me. If you feel bad, I may try to make you feel better because I feel bad about your sadness. And if I think you are making a bad decision, I will make it my mission to convince you to make a different one. Not for your sake, for mine.

If, however, you listen to a friend without thinking or worrying about how what they're saying will affect you, or planning what you might say next, that listening will open up a whole new perspective. Your friend may feel heard in a way they had not experienced before, and the connection between you is bound to strengthen. This is the beginning of a true relationship, which is built on shared mindfulness and shared presence, rather than shared opinions.

In some ways, this is the end of relationships as we know them, because it turns the act of relating into a present moment activity. A relationship becomes a sharing of life now rather than a sharing of history. This has become my experience over the past few years, and it has added incredible depth to my relationships with other humans. I find that I fall in love with almost every person I meet almost immediately. After a five-minute interaction, I smile when I remember them, and I feel a warmth that doesn't want anything from them. The same goes for mindful friends who email me from around the world. I have a deep sense of care for them and I hope they will wake up into peace and happiness, even though I may never meet them. At the same time, I could peacefully say goodbye to anyone in my life without the intense sadness I would have experienced a few years ago. There is less attachment, but more openness, more care and love. Here is a simple way to experience a taste of this:

Activity: Mr Right Now

The popular saying goes that you should wait for Mr Right, not just Mr Right Now. Let's flip this on its head today (though not in a romantic way!). Today, treat whoever you are with as the most important person in the world while you are with them. Listen intently to what they say, pay close attention to their posture, their face and their tone of voice. Give this person your full attention, until they or you move on. Repeat this process throughout the day, and notice if the way you experience those people changes. You may be surprised with the results when you focus on Mr (or Mrs) Right Now.

When doing this, I find it helpful to feel my breath while listening, as it helps me to stay present with the person I am with. You may find this useful too.

Enjoy those instantaneous relationships today and notice how your world starts to change. Moving from thought-based, historical relationships to relating through fresh, joyful aliveness is a wonderful way to live.

Finally, when you are free of judgements, you can be wholehearted in your actions, which brings a sense of calm, peace and joy. It also makes you increasingly effective because old beliefs, assumptions and conditioning no longer contaminate your actions in this moment.

Day 3: The End of Worry

Future Focus

No matter what area of life you are focusing on, it is normal for us humans to be worried, stressed and anxious when we think about the future. This may seem normal, but we can use the practice of instantaneous breathing to bring us into the present moment. And once we are in that space, instantaneous focus has some powerful applications for day-to-day life. One place we can use this skill is in difficult situations. The thing that's stressful about a challenge in life is not the situation itself. What is stressful is the act of thinking about the situation. It's the thoughts that are scary (if we believe them), and when we get lost in those thoughts, fear and anxiety are almost inevitable.

Most people worry about work not when they are working, but when they are safely tucked into their nice warm beds. After all, worry is by nature a future-focused activity. It is impossible to worry about what is; we can only worry about what might happen in the future (which never comes because it keeps turning into the present).

As a simple example, when you're sick, your mind may start projecting that you're going to miss work, your boss is going to be upset, you're not going to be able to go on your holiday, or maybe you're actually going to die – this illness is going to kill you. What's distressing you is not the illness – it's the fear of what will happen because of the illness.

A similar example is money, which is something a lot people worry about, and something I have spent plenty of time worrying about myself. But the worry is very rarely about Now. The fear is that I won't be able to afford this, or I won't be able to do that, or I'm not going to be able to pay the rent or afford food next week. Although these are challenging situations, the fear is about the future, because when you get to the spot where you can't pay, there is nothing to worry about any more: it has already happened.

All you really need to do is pay attention to one part of your life: this instant. Rather than worrying about the whole thing or what might happen next – rather than trying to deal with the imaginary – just deal with the fact: right now I am sick. My body is sick, and I need to rest. I am going to bed now. I am not coming into work, I am turning off my phone, and I am resting. I am going to let the body take care of what happens next.

Now if I wake up and I'm still not feeling better, I might decide to take some other action. I might take some medicine, I might go to see a doctor, or I might stick my head over a steaming bowl of water – whatever is needed. I make that decision, or that decision makes itself, and I act and then leave it behind, just like the last breath. I just leave it behind. I keep walking this razor's edge of Now, staying with this exact piece, this exact instant of my experience – the only instant that exists – which is Now.

You are no longer worrying about the next Now or the last Now. It is just this; it is all just this. And suddenly difficult situations aren't difficult any more. They are just challenges that either require action or don't. If they require action, you act, and if not, you leave it – very simple. The mind will try to complicate this and say, 'Yeah, but ... what about ... what if ...', but there is no situation where being in the Now doesn't apply. In any situation, all you can do is act in the best way you can, or not act. There is no other path or option. When you keep this in mind, life is very simple.

Then what happens to worry? It dissolves. And as it dissolves, the energy you were spending on futile worrying becomes free to be used in your action now. It's as if you had millions of pounds that you kept throwing down a well, planning for the future, but leaving barely enough for you to enjoy this moment. This is how the mind operates: as if the future were more important than what is. So when you stop throwing money down the well, that energy is yours. And when you spend that energy in the one place and time you can actually do some good, you will be a blessing to those around you.

Ending worry is as simple as that! Every time it arises, take attention from the thoughts about the future and place it on the present moment's activities. And as worry dissolves, that energy is yours to spend as you wish!

Activity: Turning Worry into Power

Consider an activity, a relationship or a situation in which you spend a great deal of energy pre-planning and worrying. This might be something you avoid, like completing your tax return, a situation you find challenging, like having a difficult conversation with a work colleague, or spending time with someone you try to avoid (at family gatherings perhaps). When you think back on the days and weeks leading up to this event, how much time and energy did you invest in pre-worrying? How many hours or days did you spend imagining what might happen and mentally preparing for it? And what was the return on that investment? Did you deal with the situation any better than you could have done with minimal pre-planning? Or was it more difficult because of your elevated heart rate, sweaty palms and racing thoughts just beforehand?

Be honest with yourself and consider this alternative: think of something you're anticipating now, something that you're expecting in the next week and which is consuming some of your time and energy. For the next 24 hours, every time you find yourself devoting energy to that worry, take a mindful breath and return your attention to whatever you are doing at this instant. As you do so, notice how your experience of life changes when you are primarily focused on life as it is in this instant.

Day 4: Working on the Razor's Edge

A Means to an End

In the world of work, most of us follow the usual approach, that is, we look to the past as an authority, using this information to decide what we need to do now to get us to the perfect future. Whatever you want from work, be it money, prestige, status or a warm fuzzy feeling, work can easily become a means to an end. And as soon as any pursuit becomes a means to get somewhere, the joy of the activity is lost, as is our attention to detail, our focus on the activity itself. It seems counter-intuitive, but the less you think about the future, the better it will be. If you stop worrying about your future success and pay close attention to the work you are doing now, you will find yourself more productive, creative and calm at work. You will achieve more with less stress, in less time and will discover creative ideas to help your company along the way. Does this sound like the type of employee who needs to worry about their future? Calm, clear, efficient work is the best possible career move. As a bonus, being focused on the work you are doing now makes the process of working far more enjoyable, regardless of what that work is.

I believe this is why many people love hobbies, many of which are as mundane and repetitive as the work they do, because when knitting, or gardening, there is not much thought of what I want to get from this. Wanting pollutes the pure joy of activity, while pure activity is joyful, whether the world considers it mundane or exciting.

So what is your work – an expression of joyful activity or a struggle to get somewhere? The answer to this question determines not just your enjoyment of your work, but also your contribution to the world while you are working. This may sound grand, but we contribute to the world all the time, we contribute energy. It could be gruff, complaining, bitter energy or it could be the pure joy of enthusiasm, either way it's a contribution. A waiter or a bank clerk can contribute just as much – as you will know if you have been served by someone who exudes joy and friendliness in everything they do – as a heart surgeon, though they may not get the same recognition. Whatever you are doing today, you are adding something to the world, and it's up to you what that contribution is.

As I write these words, I know that if I try to get them done as quickly as possible, two things will happen: firstly, my work will suffer, and secondly you will enjoy these words less. As I write each word for its own sake, it is joyful, although it looks ordinary. I can almost sense you reading these words and I hope you can taste the attention, the awareness out of which they arise. It is that awareness that is doing, is writing, much better than my mind ever could. My mind wants the job done, so it can never linger over the quality, the enjoyment of the act of writing.

And so when I go to work during the day in social welfare, there are many tasks to complete, many jobs to be done, people to serve. There too I can either stay focused on getting through the list, or I can delight in each instant, regardless of what it calls for. If it calls for administration, statistical analysis and checking emails, I love it. If it calls for sitting and talking with clients, I love that too. I love these activities not because of the activities, but because I love being present, I love being awake. And you will too.

Activity: One Thing at a Time

When you go to work (or study or whatever regular activity you do) today, take a different approach, act as if you have no future, as if this instant, this task is your entire life. Act as if you had chosen to do this task, this job, and as if time has no reality. Then, simply complete each task with care and attention before moving on to the next thing (which is always 'this thing' really. Have you ever done 'the next thing'?). There is no need to take extra time to do tasks, nor do you need to be silent, still and contemplative. Do what you usually do, but with careful attention to detail.

When I work with this sort of present-moment focus, I notice three interesting changes. Firstly, my work improves, because I am careful and attentive. Secondly, I feel calm and peaceful, and those around me become peaceful too. And finally (and most surprisingly), I get better at planning for the future and executing plans, achieving goals. This surprised me at first, but it makes perfect sense. When you are clear, you know what to do next and how to work through a plan. You also bring enough attention to stay with the plan until it is complete. Contrary to what the mind may say, instantaneous work is the way of peace, quality and productivity.

Take note of what happens for you when you work with this present-moment focus.

Day 5: The Source of Creativity

Repetitive Thinking

Have you ever had a moment of brilliance, a flash of inspiration? What if you could be in a state of consciousness that invited this brilliance, this creativity to express itself, every day? Well you can, but first we need to understand where this creative spark arises from and why it is so rare for most people.

As you will have noticed by now, most people live almost entirely lost in thought, consumed in the stories of the mind. People churn over the same old thoughts day after day, year after year, the same soap operas consuming their energy and attention. And without energy and attention to spare, would you expect the fiery spark that is creativity to be able to arise? No way. For that, we need the freshness, the vitality of the present moment.

The mind has no interest in the present moment; in fact, it is incapable of being present. Instead, the mind studies the past, believing that if it understands the past, it can eliminate the bad and increase the good, thereby achieving happiness in the future. If you have read Eckhart Tolle's work, you will be familiar with the concept of using the present moment as a means to an end – the belief that happiness or salvation (as some people call it) is somehow going to arise in the future, and the quicker we get to that future, the quicker we will find happiness.

Therefore, our minds continually analyse the past, scanning for everything that went wrong – everything that should have been different – and trying to figure out how to change it in the future, so that we can be happy. We have a belief that once all our ducks are in a row, once we've got everything figured out and set up perfectly, then we will be happy, then we will find peace. Of course, the unfortunate truth is that it's the process of chasing that future happiness that keeps dragging our attention away from the happiness that's already here, inside us right now.

So, of course, we end up stressed, striving for future happiness. And how could creativity co-exist with stress? Creativity is playful, unconcerned with progress, it creates for the fun of it. Stress is its opposite. If we combine stress with the constant regurgitation of the same old thoughts and stories, which leaves no room for anything new to enter this world, what chance does that creative spark have of lighting a fire underneath you? Almost none.

As it stands today, creativity has to sneak into most people's worlds. It has to jump through a gap when you finally get tired and stop thinking for a moment, or when you are so challenged that those old thoughts lose their place as the centre of attention. How many times has the answer come to you when you were engaged in some unrelated activity, in the shower, in the garden, or when you stepped away to take a break? Exhausted from trying to figure it out, the mind stops thinking about it and the fresh, unexpected answer exposes itself, boom!

This happens to me every single day. Take note that I say it happens to me, I don't say that I am creative or that I do it, it just happens. When I talk to my supervisor at work I often say, 'I had a crazy idea' and she smiles, because she knows something fresh and new is arising, not from me but from the creative energy of the universe. After all, the energy of the universe has created trillions of different life forms, and those forms continue to evolve with unfathomable intelligence. If I allow just a little of that energy into my life, then of course it can solve the petty problems my mind would love to chew on for a few thousand years! And minds do love problems, much more than solutions.

Your mind fears the solution, because if all problems were solved, it would have nothing to do! Try giving someone a simple solution to a problem they are deeply attached to and you will see the fear arise. They may even attack you and your solution! To unleash your creativity, you must sidestep the mind!

Activity: Sidestepping the Mind

Today I want to invite you into a different way of living this life, as a form of play, by stepping into the flow of creativity. This is a process I stumbled on by accident, and I use it every day to bring a little more joy and freshness into my world.

Start by making a list of five playful activities you enjoy. Playful activities must be things you do without trying to achieve anything or get anywhere in particular, like dancing, singing or doing a handstand! Once you have made your list, pick an activity to do today. Set a timer for 15 minutes (no interruptions allowed unless the house catches on fire) and enjoy! Do the activity the way a five-year-old would, with no consideration that something else might be a better use of your time.

Allow your attention to stay with the activity, let any other thoughts come and go, but keep focused on your play as much as you can.

Once the timer sounds, leave the activity if you wish (or keep going if you're hooked) and continue with your day. Bring this same focused, playful energy into the rest of your day's activities and see what happens next!

If you spend 15 minutes each day playing, your spark will ignite and creativity will find another channel to flow into this world. And this is a wonderful thing.

Day 6: Mindful Past, Skilful Future

Mindful Planning

It might seem odd that a practice that denies the reality of time can improve mental abilities like memory, thinking and cognitive processing. Yet you will find that when you sharpen your focus to this instant of your life, your ability to remember and learn from the past will flourish, as will your skill in anticipating and planning for the future. Of course, the future doesn't really exist, it's just that this Now changes shape, so I prefer to call it 'the next change' instead of 'the future'. Either way, there is a certain skilfulness in planning and learning that arises when you are present, right here and now.

Ice Hockey champion Wayne Gretzky was by far the greatest of all time in his field, and was well known for his ability to anticipate where the puck would end up next. Far from the fastest skater, he was instead the best reader of the present moment. I would confidently guess that when Mr Gretzky was on the ice, he was intently focused on the present moment, completely alert and aware in the instant. When you spend long periods of time engaged in an activity in this state, you begin to see the patterns and learn to read the next move required. And we can all live like this.

This type of approach is quite different from the usual way, because it is not a thinking process (although thought may be involved). It is a process of watching closely and responding almost instinctively to what arises now. Driving your car with careful attention is an example of this. Over years, you learn to anticipate what other cars may do, how the curve of the road may affect your steering and how hard to brake. As you drive, there is no need to think about what you are doing (which is why so many people daydream from A to B), but if you stay alert and focused, you will find that skilful, safe driving happens quite naturally, and that it is quite enjoyable. This can easily be applied to whatever you do on a day-to-day basis, but you have to be present.

Lost in thought, it is very difficult to learn from this moment, because we already know. We know what is best, what should be and what's wrong with this moment, and these judgements cut us off from the ability to watch, listen and learn. Observe the next time you start judging another driver on the road, and see how this reduces your awareness of what you are doing. Lost in the fog of the mind, most humans are only dimly aware of what is happening around them because there is so much noise going on inside them instead! The following exercise shows a different way, an approach to being mentally sharp every single day.

Activity: Mindful Remembering, Skilful Planning

Take a moment to remember a difficult experience from the past few weeks. Pick something that was challenging, but that isn't a source of serious pain or trauma. Take a few minutes to look back on that experience or event, and feel yourself breathing at the same time. Don't try to gain anything or learn anything, just breathe and reflect, and allow any insights or learnings to arise by themselves.

Now bring to mind something you would like to do in the coming weeks, like a project, a trip or an excursion somewhere. Rather than agonising over what you will do and what might go wrong, sit, breathe and allow the idea of that activity to sit with you. Take a few minutes to enjoy the process of breathing and sitting with an idea, a plan that isn't yet formed. Allow any insights about how you might approach this activity to bubble to the surface and don't worry if they don't, just sit and enjoy.

This is my way of planning and learning from the past and I have found some surprising results. Plans make themselves when I allow them to and past learnings bubble away without any effort. Because of this, I learn and improve more than ever before in my life, and my approach to work, personal life, just life really, is virtually unflappable. And it feels so peaceful.

The world has taught us that stress and hard work are the way to improve things, but practise these skills this week and you may well find that the opposite is true.

Day 7: Living Mindfully: From thinking to experience

How was Your Day?

We have been conditioned to pay more attention to our thoughts than to our experience, as if opinions and judgements were somehow more reliable than the actual experience of living. When you tell someone how your day was, you don't talk about the actual experience of the sunshine or the wind or the rain, or the feeling of sitting in your chair at your desk, or the sound of the voices around you. What you talk about is your thoughts about your day: 'That person was too bossy; I didn't get paid enough; it was too cold (or too hot); I hate my job ...' That is what you were paying attention to. Rather than asking how someone's day was, it would be much more accurate to ask, 'How was your thinking today?'

But you have an opportunity to step out of that thought-based existence – an existence that becomes appalling once you've experienced something different. You have an opportunity to shift into experiential existence, which is really existing, really living and really enjoying even the simplest things. You will make a shift of the highest order. But how?

Start Noticing

Experiencing life as it happens is not possible through the mind – it is only possible by stepping out of thinking and into curiosity and openness. Thoughts are constantly describing, labelling, judging, and measuring the world around us. They act as the experts on the state of the world – on what is good, bad or ugly – and they tell us how we should feel, react and behave in response to events.

This position of expertise means that thoughts are closed; they have a firm, fixed view of the world based on their knowledge and their version of truth. Unfortunately, when you think you know, you immediately stop looking and stop experiencing things directly. This is the curse of the expert.

When we stop thinking about the world and start noticing, however, openness and curiosity become natural. When you look without getting lost in thought, you experience a totally different world. Try this experiment in a familiar environment like your home or workplace: take five minutes to walk around and take in as much about your surroundings as you can without getting lost in thoughts. Follow your breath and just look, as if you had never been there before.

You will be amazed how many previously unnoticed details become evident when you look without judging. You will possibly even learn that you know very little directly about this place, despite spending so much time there. You may find, in fact, that your time there is really spent in your head! Extend this experiment to the people around you, and you will notice some amazing shifts in the quality of your relationships.

To become instantaneously focused, the first thing you need to do is find the breath. As you learn to pay attention to the breath, you shift from thinking to experience. You can make that shift now by taking your attention inside your body.

Activity: Just This Breath

Notice how it feels as you breathe in, and as you breathe out. Feel what it's like to breathe. We all know that we breathe (we're at least dimly aware of it), but for the next few moments, bring your focus intently to the in-breath and to the out-breath.

And as you do so, keep honing your focus – keep sharpening your awareness down and down and down – until you are focused on just this one breath. Don't worry about the next breath. And as soon as the last breath is gone, forget it by moving on to this breath – always this breath. Feel this in-breath, feel this out-breath, and so on.

At the end of each in-breath and each out-breath, check where your attention is. Are you lost in a thought? Or are you aware, right here and now? Follow this in-breath and check yourself – where are you? Follow this out-breath and check yourself again – where are you? As you do that, continue to sharpen your focus so that you are following just this one part of this breath. You are not even worried about the whole breath; your awareness is intently focused on this one part, this one section, of this breath.

You will notice a slight pause between breaths, perhaps after the out-breath. When that pause comes, sit in it and use it to check yourself and refocus. Follow this in-breath, instant by instant; follow this out-breath, instant by instant; and check yourself in the pause. Keep coming back – now this breath, now this breath, now this breath – always now, now, now, now.

This probably sounds very simple. But if you're trying to do it, or if you have tried before, you will know that it's not. Although there's nothing complicated about it, the mind is complicated. Doing something simple is really hard because your mind wants to go off in all sorts of interesting directions, and it wants to take you with it.

Practising Instantaneous Focus

This first shift you'll make on your journey will bring greater intensity, excitement and interest to your life. I encourage you to bring your curiosity to it, to be really open to what you experience, regardless of what your mind says.

It becomes more intense, more interesting and more exciting as we start to notice what's around us instead of thinking about what's next. We start to notice the colours, sounds and shapes, and we start to really experience our lives as they are happening rather than always living through the fog of the mind – always looking to the next thing, always valuing what comes next over what is right now.

Finally, remember that this is not just a book – it's a course – and the free downloads available on the website are there to support you on your journey. You can find them at www.olidoyle.com/MFL.

WEEK 2

Allowfulness

To find real peace, you will have to make peace with your inner world. The outer world is another story – but you will discover that when you are in accord with the inner world, the outer seems much more pleasant. So we work with the inner, and we either enjoy the outer or use it as fuel for our practice. To do this, we will focus this week on learning the skill I call 'allowfulness', which begins with a journey of curiosity into our thoughts and emotions.

Allowfulness is a word that came into my mind one day as a way to describe what seems to be a paradox: accepting what is while simultaneously acting to improve it. Allowfulness means allowing this moment to be exactly as it is, and then doing what you can to make a positive change. It frees us from many of the habits of humans that are energy sapping, destructive and largely pointless – habits that aim to control the way life unfolds.

What we will learn this week is how to break out of that cycle, how to do something radically different, how to instead dive into those feelings in a way that is safe. We will learn how to embrace whatever arises internally and externally – and to then do whatever we can to improve it.

The Myth of Progress

A lot of people who practise mindfulness get caught up in the notion that this practice is linear. 'I need to do it right, I need to do it well and then I am a good meditator,' and so on. 'I am getting closer to enlightenment. I will get there soon … faster than you' or 'I am a terrible student. I can't do this. Why should I bother? I will never sit again. I am going to turn the TV back on. I will never get to enlightenment, or everyone else will get there first. They will have eaten all the good food by the time I get there.' (This was certainly me in my first five years of practice.)

But this practice is not linear. There is no place that we are trying to get to. We are just practising being present in this moment. There can be no future destination because future means thinking, and mindfulness is the art of learning not to think. Of course, thought still arises, but we learn to stop fussing with thoughts, stressing about them and playing with them. We learn to sit and watch instead.

So this week, be careful that your mind does not turn the practice of allowfulness into a way to make progress, a way to stop the power of pain and suffering. This progress implies future, the pursuit of which is causing your suffering in the first place. Take progress off the table this week, and instead learn to allow this moment (and yourself) to be just as it is.

Day 1: Allow Yourself

Arguing with Myself

Most humans are not entirely happy with who they are. They believe themselves to be too old, too heavy, too pale, too poor, or some other variation on this theme. Of course, these stories are not reality, they are just stories, thoughts repeated in the mind and believed. The mind uses these stories to try to motivate us to be better, faster, healthier, smarter, but the result is simply pain, and perhaps a combination of the behaviours we are seeking to change. In truth, the mind, exposed to anything for long enough, will find something to complain about, and you are no different. It is an expert at finding what is lacking, or what is in excess, and making that into a problem. Before we explore this further I want to be clear: I am not saying that you should not try to improve your health, your job prospects or anything else about your life, but I also want to be clear about the cost of turning yourself into a walking problem.

I also want to be crystal clear about the reality of your life this instant: it is exactly as it is. This isn't the most profound revelation perhaps, but consider this: whether you beat yourself up or not, you are exactly as you are in this instant. Would you rather be exactly as you are and at peace with yourself, or at war? This is the only choice.

As it turns out, people who are at peace with themselves as they are seem to make better choices about taking care of this body and this life. After all, did all that guilt about your weight ever lead to a healthy lifestyle in the long term? Did the gnawing anxiety about some impulse buy make you a responsible money manager? Or did these feelings of negativity and low self-worth merely feed the cycle that leads to those behaviours in the first place? And what was the cost, in time, energy and stress, of all that self-criticism?

The flawed assumption underneath this cycle, of course, is that self-criticism will lead to self-improvement, which will lead (eventually) to future happiness. But as the only moment you will ever experience is this one, happiness can only be here now. And as we have seen already, the very source of dissatisfaction is the act of looking to the future for fulfilment. If you live by this pattern, you will never find happiness or self-acceptance, because as soon as you arrive at the place the mind says you 'should' be at, be it a particular weight, salary or something else, your goals will shift. You have no doubt experienced this phenomenon, when you thought that a new car would lead to happiness, but after a few weeks of owning it you started thinking how run-down your house was, and so it goes on. The same applies to your story of yourself. Even if you arrive at the perfect point in terms of health, wealth, relationships and everything else, there will soon enough be a downward slide as death approaches. This is the fatal flaw in looking for contentment by changing something about you or the world: it always fails eventually. Let's try something different.

So, what happened there? Nothing about you improved, but perhaps you were able to enjoy yourself, even for a moment or two. The reason for this is that, I hope, you stepped out of story for a brief moment, and this is the key to being content within yourself. When you step out of story, you find the place in you that is already content, the part that can't be improved: pure awareness. And from there you can enjoy watching the game of life, the coming and going. One of the names for

Buddha is Tathagata, which roughly translates as 'looks like coming, looks like going'. Isn't that beautiful? Everything about me looks like coming, looks like going; it is arising or disappearing in each instant. As breath comes and goes, we can learn how to live skilfully when it comes to improving ourselves. When wealth comes, enjoy it; when it goes, enjoy that. When health comes, enjoy it, and when it goes, let it (it will anyway). In this way, holding our so-called achievements and our so-called failures lightly, we learn to appreciate what exists beyond both, which is your life this instant. No story, no worries.

Activity: Allowing Yourself

Today I invite you to explore what happens when, instead of looking to chisel, shape and change yourself, you enjoy yourself as you are this instant. Close your eyes for a moment once you have read these instructions and take your attention to your breath. Feel the air coming and going, feel how the body moves and changes with each in- and out-breath, and let each breath be exactly as long or short as it is. Allow the breath to come and go, and allow yourself to rest on it, enjoy the feeling of coming and going. Sit with this for a few minutes, and whenever the mind comes in with something you need to do, achieve or think about, come back to enjoying yourself, exactly as you are. And after you stand up and move on with the day, remember that this pure simple enjoyment is with you, always.

Day 2: Peaceful Relationships

From Judgement to Curiosity

When we practise allowfulness, we are moving from thought to experience. We also need to move from judgement to curiosity. This entails a similar process of going from thinking we know what should happen and what's best for us in the world, to being curious about what happens, being interested in it and wondering about it, rather than having a closed mind. As soon as we think we know, we stop looking (all good scientists know this), and it is the looking itself that brings us into the present moment. It is looking with fresh eyes every time. The move from judgement to curiosity is really an opening – a shifting of the mind from a closed position to a wondering position.

On a practical level, this gives us a wider scope for living effectively. We all know people who are stuck in thinking they know everything. It becomes really hard for people like that to learn new things or develop truly loving relationships. Love is not about romance or giving people things or even being nice to people; true love is about being completely present and allowing people to be exactly as they are.

It is impossible to do this from a place of judgement, which is why making the shift to curiosity has such a powerful effect on relationships. That shift also eliminates a whole lot of stress, because much of our stress comes from judgements about people and situations. 'I should have more money. People should appreciate me. People should be nice to me' – and so on and so forth.

When we think we know what's best, we get lost in those

thoughts over and over again, and it creates stress. The stress isn't caused by not having enough money; the stress comes from thinking about the money that you don't have or that you should have. You can be poor and peaceful, or you can be rich and stressed – we all know that. And when it comes to relationships, you can be single and happy, or in a relationship and miserable. There is a simple cause for this misery, and it is called wanting. You want your partner (or your friend, your mother, your boss, it's all the same) to be more loving. You want them to appreciate you, and perhaps more than anything you want their approval. And when we have so many wants, what is happening when we are in front of another human being, having a conversation or a cup of tea? Thinking.

'What did she mean when she said ...? Does she still like me? I can't tell any more ... Did he really like that gift, or was he pretending?'

When you sit in front of me and I am lost in thought, I don't see you, I don't hear you, I'm too busy thinking about me. 'What does that statement mean for me? What does it mean if you like me, or hate me? And what should I do next to make you like me a little bit more?' Of course, these thoughts aren't usually so conscious or transparent, but examine your words, your feelings and your actions and you will find them!

What if we could sit together and have that same conversation, without either of us caring what the other one thought? I wouldn't need to try to be witty or act compassionate unless it spontaneously arose, and you could just listen and enjoy what I was saying, without needing to influence my mental life. It sounds lovely, doesn't it?

Perhaps you have a relationship like this with a friend,

someone who you know won't judge you, no matter what you say. When you relax and sit with someone in this state of allowfulness, it is absolutely divine and, in truth, every interaction you have can be like this.

Activity: Interested in You

To experience this way of being with others, try this during a conversation you have today: completely suspend your own interests. Act as if you are speaking with the most interesting, important person in the world and become totally absorbed in what they say, in their thoughts, feelings, ideas and experiences. Become like a skilled interviewer, soaking up what the other says with no care for your own opinions. See if you can listen without needing to judge or analyse what is being said, just listen completely, absorb it and allow your response to arise naturally.

Notice the urge to but in, to tell your own story, to take the conversation in another direction, and when that urge arises, come back to listening and see what happens next.

In reality, the person in front of you now (regardless of your story about them) is the most important person in your world. In fact, they're the only one! When you learn to treat people with this level of curiosity, something amazing happens: you become a friend of whoever you are with right now, and as a side benefit, relationships with everyone you meet become loving and enjoyable. Of course, there will still be people in your life who you are drawn to, and others with whom you don't resonate, but in the moment of interaction, you can treat each person in the same way.

As an experiment this week, I invite you to treat close friends and family with this level of curiosity and to notice how those relationships start to change.

Day 3: Let It Be (As It Is)

Working with Emotions

We humans also spend a lot of time and energy warring with our own internal states. We spend our precious internal resources trying to change our anger, trying to get rid of our sadness, trying to escape from our anxiety.

We argue with reality outside and with our feelings inside. When it comes to the internal world, our battles can take on epic proportions. Our normal way of dealing with unpleasant emotions is to get rid of them, to change them, to suppress them or to ignore them. That is what we are taught, and that is what most of us do most of the time. There are two consequences of this: first, we become afraid of feelings and we avoid them. I would certainly argue that as the 21st century rolls on, humans are becoming less and less tolerant of painful feelings. We are giving credence to the expectation that we should feel good most of the time. And we have a lot of tools for doing that, even when our internal state makes it difficult to feel good naturally.

The second thing that happens when we try to control our feelings is that they grow. They get stronger and they multiply. Anything you fight gains energy from the fight; anything you resist or try to get rid of tends to cling more tightly. For example, when you try to get rid of your anger, you may find yourself becoming angry that you can't make it go away, or angry that it is there in the first place, and so anger grows. You may feel sad about wasting so much energy on anger, and so sadness joins the party. You may feel guilty about wasting so much time on emotions that do nothing for you, and so guilt comes along to play as well. The emotions grow and grow.

As we keep fighting and losing these battles, we slip more and more into the world of story, and in this half-life, there is so much pain, so much discomfort, so much unhappiness and dissatisfaction, because we know deep down what we are capable of. We know what we deserve and what we were born for. Yet we find ourselves lost in this world, half-asleep and half-awake.

To discover the peace that each of us is capable of, we must learn to practise allowfulness.

The best way to learn allowfulness, in my opinion, is to spend time with difficult feelings, because this is usually the area that's most problematic for us, and it's the place we want to escape from quickly. But it's also an area that provides frequent opportunities for practice, because difficult feelings tend to arise every day for most of us.

Today's practice is going to centre around something really simple: tension or stress in the body. You are likely to be carrying some tension and stress right now in your muscles or joints or even your organs. Today I invite you to do the opposite of what the world has taught you, to practise diving into the tension and stress, really exploring it, and being OK with it. In doing that, you will gradually build your ability to allow. You will build your ability to observe, notice and sit curiously with what is – without getting caught up in the stories that the mind tells about reality.

Activity: Practising Allowfulness

As you are sitting there reading this, take your attention inside and notice what it feels like as the breath comes and goes. Notice those physical sensations. Take a few minutes to feel your body as a whole. See whether you can feel your entire body at once, and as you are doing so, try to notice where in the body you are carrying stress or feeling tension. You don't need to worry about why it's there; you don't need to think about the situations that caused it or what you need to do about those situations. You just need to fully experience and explore those sensations.

Notice what the stress feels like as a physical sensation in the body right now. Take your attention into it and notice what type of sensation it is. Feel the emotion as a physical sensation, the way you would feel a headache or a sore finger. Notice how it moves or doesn't. Notice the weight of it, the texture of it and the size of it. Notice those things, not to catalogue them or better understand them, but just as a way to stay curious, to keep sparking your interest and openness. Keep coming back to the sensation; keep feeling it.

As you do, be watchful for the mind's attempts to hijack your attention and take your awareness somewhere else – into a thought or a story about why the stress is there and what to do about it, or a story about what is wrong in your life and what you need to change. Whenever that happens, come back to the direct experience instead.

Allowing the Sensations

Keep coming back whenever your mind takes you somewhere else. Whenever you want to escape, return to allowing
the sensation to be as it is for this instant, for this second.
You don't have to allow it a second longer than that – just for
this second. And after this second goes, allow it for this second. Make friends with the emotion or sensation. You don't
need to build a big story around it. You can simply experience it. Feel it, sit with it and allow it to be there.

You are doing something really important here. You are
stepping out of story and into experience. You are allowing
the body to process the stress in its own time, and you are giving it the space to do so. You are also building your ability to
be with difficulty, challenges and discomfort; you are breaking the cycle of pain.

Breaking the Cycle of Pain

As you master this practice, you are learning to break the
link between feelings and thoughts. Ordinarily, when negative feelings like stress or anxiety arise, our thoughts feed
those feelings. And as we get lost in the thoughts, the feelings
get stronger. The more the feelings grow, the stronger the
thoughts become. As that snowball continues, the thoughts
and feelings get bigger and bigger and more and more overwhelming.

For example, if your partner or friend snaps at you, you
might feel angry when you think about it later. There you are,

cooking dinner or reading a book, when suddenly the memory of that snapping arises, and anger quickly follows. As the anger builds, it feeds the story of what happened, what you should have said or done in response, and what you need to do next. In other words, you re-imagine the past and project the future. As that story rolls on, the anger gets stronger, which feeds the story, and the cycle continues.

When we practise allowfulness, what we are doing instead is taking a step back whenever the thoughts start to take over. We return to experiencing the feeling as it is – as a physical sensation. That's it. If you can learn to do that, you will never have an emotional problem again. When the emotion tries to take over your thinking, or vice versa, you can sit and experience the feeling while watching the thoughts roll by. It's as if you were sitting in a nice warm house watching a thunderstorm roll through: beautiful, powerful and unable to stop your happiness.

Using Resistance as Fuel for Mindfulness

Embrace these areas of resistance and suddenly finding those places of stuckness becomes a celebration of the growing recognition and awareness that you are not your mind, that thought is not everything, and that the mind doesn't know it all. You can begin to use every experience to deepen your contact with the present moment.

Feelings of anger, rather than being a problem, become something you can pay attention to, something you can dive into. You no longer need to change or do anything with your anger; you can just be mindful of it. If you experience great sadness, then sadness becomes your practice.

This does something really important and interesting: it takes away the fear of those feelings and the fear of not being a good enough mindfulness practitioner. The fear itself is part of your practice and something you can make friends with. In allowfulness, there is nothing we exclude – nothing.

Day 4: Allowfulness at Work

Making Peace with Your Job

As we walk through this world as human beings, we tend to get into struggles with life. We engage in battles that we can't win – battles to change the past or control the future. We get lost in endless scheming, planning, manipulating and even tantrums in our vain attempts to do the impossible – to change the way the world looks right now.

Take a look around you and tell me this: can you change the way your surroundings look at the moment? I don't mean in five seconds from now, or in ten years, but can you change how things appear now? Can you change your emotions, your thoughts or the state of your body in this instant? And can you change your financial situation, your relationships or your workplace in this very moment? If you are honest, the answer is no. Of course, you can take action now and that may lead to change, but as each instant unfolds, it is exactly as it is, without exception. When you argue with reality, you inevitably lose.

One place in which this argument is strong for many people is their place of work, their place of service. I prefer the term service because it covers whatever you do on a day-to-day basis, be it paid work, raising a family, caring for others or looking for paid work. Whatever that daily ritual is, many humans find that their mind is not particularly happy with it. Perhaps the work is repetitive, perhaps it is poorly paid or unpaid, and perhaps it appears that your contribution is unappreciated. Whatever the apparent cause, minds love to complain about this, they love to figure out what *should* be happening and compare it to what is. And this is two things: stressful and hopeless.

For one thing, reality doesn't care about your preferences. Reality just is. Second, arguing with what is only increases your frustration and draws you deeper into the world of thought, thereby strengthening the patterns that created your present moment. And finally, this argument turns life into a battleground in which it's Me vs the world, as I fight to get this moment to look the way I think it should or to get what I think I deserve. This existence is stressful, not because of the world, but because I believe I know what the world should look like, so I am at war with it.

This war is a choice you don't have to make. Instead you can allow. What if, just for a week, you stopped mentally complaining about work. What if, instead, you engaged with it fully, and tried to improve things as best you could. Mentally complaining is not an attempt to improve things, complaining is an addiction. The mind loves to complain, especially about things that are unlikely to change. It gives the mind energy, attention and something to think about: the perfect combination. But instead of repeating this useless pattern, you have the power to put that energy into improving things. First, though, you must allow them to be as they are.

Activity: Being at Peace at Work

Today I invite you to try two things that may not seem to fit together: allow work to be as it is, and do whatever you can to improve it. To do this, you must first enter the present moment with your awareness.

Bring attention to the breath for a moment and enter this now. As you do so, look around and let everything in your vision be as it is. Just look, and if judgements arise, allow them to come and go, and make the act of looking your primary focus. As you look around, you may find yourself drawn to take some action. If you're at home you may find yourself wiping crumbs off the kitchen table, if you're outside you may find yourself picking up some rubbish. Whatever you feel drawn to do, take that action with awareness and allowfulness. Stories may try to take over, perhaps about who should have wiped the table or that people should not litter, but stay with what is. The crumbs are there, and you are there, peacefully wiping the table. If there is nothing to do, then just sit and enjoy this instant.

When you go to work today, take this same attitude and see what happens. Make friends with this instant and notice what you are called to do. This is the path of peace at work, and in life.

You may be surprised at what changes when you bring allow-fulness into your place of service. Things may change, you may find yourself leaving or you might enjoy it a whole lot more. And whatever does or does not change, you can know that through you, a little more peace is entering this world.

Day 5: Letting Sparks Fly

Embracing the Mystery

Could it be that knowing is what blocks creative energy? Knowing what will happen, why it won't work, or how it should look? If you have ever tried to sit down and undertake a creative endeavour, you will have experienced this process. The mind already knows what should be achieved through the creative work, as well as the standard that it should meet. For example, if you have ever attempted to write a book, your mind may well have begun chattering about what others will think of your writing, how many people will or won't buy it and the reasons why people like you don't do things like this. But now that you are awake to the mind's tricks, you can approach every endeavour from a different perspective – you can embrace it as a mysterious adventure. In truth, all of life is a mystery in which we don't know what happens next. Become friends with this mystery, celebrate it even, and you will unlock your creative potential in every area of your life.

It is interesting that most experts (if you ask them) rarely come up with a stroke of genius, or if they do, they become so attached to their idea that they cannot see the possibility of there being a better way. Science is a great example, with almost every brilliant scientist you learnt about at school having turned conservative in their late careers, attacking the upstarts who challenged their theories. Even Einstein fell into this trap.

You too may find that, when you think you know what is best, your curiosity evaporates. And curiosity is the fuel of creativity. After all, there is no need to create something new if you already know the best way.

In Zen, there is a beautiful phrase describing the life path of creativity: 'Don't know, go straight.' This means in any given moment (always this moment), we look with fresh eyes, listen with sharp ears and stay free of the fog of thinking. To see the world this way, we must be able to look without filtering what we see through the lens of story. This is the same as the Zen practice of 'beginner's mind' made popular by Shunryu Suzuki, who emphasised the posture of the beginner as the way to live in the now. You will no doubt remember a time when you were engaged in learning something new, like driving, or starting a different job, and you may recall a sense of care, precision (even if you lacked technical skill) and interest in what you were learning. Compare this with the sloppy, haphazard way that most of us drive and you will see a key difference: the beginner is focused on this moment of the journey, while the expert is focused on the destination, or thinking about something else. Engaging as an eternal beginner is the way of mindful creativity, of letting sparks fly.

As we move from the expert's chair to a position of not knowing, we can fully experience this moment without getting lost in our story. When we look at thoughts curiously and examine them from a place of openness, stress can't help but drop away. Beginner's mind means looking at everything freshly, as if for the first time, every time you look, and letting go of the knowledge that most of us drag around like a heavy sack.

Of course, we still have knowledge, but it no longer needs to be burdensome or to get in the way of really seeing. Beginner's mind means that every time you look at a person, you are looking as if for the first time, as if you have never seen that person before. Certainly, we don't have to pretend that we don't know someone's name or that we have no memory of the person. But we look with fresh eyes, bringing curiosity, interest and openness to each encounter. When you think you know, you stop looking. When you are curious, you look harder, noticing details that were not evident before.

Stress ends when you step out of judgement and into curiosity. As you make contact with the world exactly as it is and let it be as it is, you stop fighting with it. You embrace it instead. That's when true excitement and true peace begin.

Activity: Don't Know, See What Happens

Look around you now with interest and curiosity about what you see. Look, breathe and sink into this moment. Allow it to be just as it is. Notice the way things slow down as you do this, how the list of things you 'have to' do disappears for a moment. Breathe, feel your body and relax into this instant. There is nothing to do, and yet you might do something at any moment. It may occur to you to stand up and get a glass of water or make a cup of tea – even though this moment is perfectly OK right now. Isn't that interesting? Things were already perfect, and then a cup of tea enters your world. How wonderful! And so we see that allowfulness does not prevent action but allows action to arise from a place of peace and tranquillity, which has the power to make you calm and effective.

It is possible, of course, that the same cup of tea is your mind's attempt to distract you from the practice, and that this cup of tea may lead you to reorganising cupboards or watching TV, instead of practising as you planned. To differentiate spontaneous action from simply getting distracted, you can ask this simple question: am I experiencing this moment fully, or am I thinking about it? If you find yourself moving towards the kettle in a state of awareness and focus, then the action is a spontaneous arising. If you find yourself thinking, 'I'll make a cup of tea first', then I suggest you sit a little longer, until that thought has drifted past.

Take a piece of paper and pen and look at it for a moment. Notice the colour of the paper, the texture, and feel your breath. Now put pen to paper and let creativity flow through you. It could come as a drawing, some words or some other form. Don't concern yourself with the end result; just be attentive to the process, like an infant making marks on a page for the first time. When you feel the creation is finished, stop and study it with that same curiosity. The mind may want to judge, critique and run down your work, but stay focused on that open, curious looking.

Congratulations, you remembered your curiosity!

The mind uses labels to block our curiosity. And while labelling may not be overt, as soon as some incident happens you can sense through your body what the mind is calling it. It is labelling it good or bad, right or wrong.

When you are listening to someone, watch how quickly the mind responds – especially if the subject is one you get emotional about or that you know a lot about. The mind is ready with a response before the other person has even finished talking. So judgements also block curiosity.

To truly experience life, we need to step beyond labels and judgements into curiosity. This allows us to naturally embrace our lives with the spirit of 'Oh, I wonder what happens next. I wonder what this is like.' It opens up the world of possibility because we can start to see things differently – we can see options and ideas – and it is also the gateway to creativity.

But most important, it is the path of peace because we are stepping out of reaction. We are stepping out of struggling with the moment. We are allowing it to be exactly as it is – just allowing – that's all. Allowing is nothing more than watching with openness and curiosity. We don't have to make an effort to feel OK about something. We just watch what is now, and what is now, and what is now.

Day 6: Dealing with Pain

Primary and Secondary Suffering

Physical pain and illness are an inevitable part of the life of any human, and many people ask how mindfulness can help when pain is present. Today we will explore the application of allowfulness when you experience an illness or during physical pain.

The first thing to notice in this area is that pain has two levels, or two causes if you will. There is the pain that life gives you, and the pain you give yourself through struggle. For example, you may remember an occasion when you had a headache but also had something important to do at the same time. You may have noticed that shifting attention from the headache to your activities made the pain seem less. On another day, with a similar headache, but with nothing to do, the pain may seem much worse, but only if you are engaged in a struggle with the pain. If you sit there all day mentally complaining about the pain, worrying about the cause of it and generally arguing with life, you will inflict mental suffering on yourself, while also making the physical pain seem more intense.

The same applies with an illness like a cold. If you stay at home worrying about the work you can't get done, or stressing about the party you might miss at the weekend, the experience is a whole lot worse. On the other hand, if you are able to sit and enjoy some rest time, even though the body may feel tired, sore or depleted, the experience is much more pleasant.

Allowing any challenging experience to be as it is provides two clear benefits: firstly it frees us from the struggle that causes secondary suffering. Secondly it makes that challenge a part of our mindfulness practice, an opportunity to step firmly into this instant with curiosity and attention. Living from that awareness is its own reward, making life enjoyable, even when pain and illness are there. The usual way to approach such situations is to judge them mentally, tell our story to others and to dwell in the injustice of the whole experience. Once again, we become the expert, who knows what life should be doing, or in the words of Eckhart Tolle, we become 'morally superior to life!' Knowing best is incredibly frustrating when life couldn't care less about our opinions. And so we have a choice to make: will we continue to oppose what is, even though that doesn't make it change, or will we consider, for an instant, that perhaps what is happening is what is meant to be happening? If we allow the second choice to be at least a possibility, we can bring a little curiosity into our internal world.

Activity: Internal Curiosity

Let's take a moment to enjoy some curious exploration of the body from the inside. This process is what I recommend any time you are sick or in pain. Close your eyes, take your attention inside and notice your breath. From there, see if you can feel your entire body and notice all the different sensations rippling through it right now. Don't become too focused on one particular sensation, stay with the entire body and enjoy the constant movement of sensations.

Whenever the mind drags you away from this process, come back and be present with the physical body right now. The mind may tell stories about pain, about discomfort or about something else, but stay sharp, stay aware and enjoy this second.

Normally, when physical suffering is there, two things happen: the mind generates large amounts of thought about the suffering and why it shouldn't be there, and we become exclusively focused on that one part of our present-moment experience. The mind is a sophisticated complaint-generation machine, but this process achieves nothing except the addition of secondary suffering to your present moment.

Instead, you may like to try this: take action to alleviate primary suffering if you can but, if you can't, allow what is.

This may or may not lessen the physical pain, but it will definitely reduce or eliminate secondary suffering and make life a whole lot more enjoyable.

And finally, pain and suffering are excellent mindfulness teachers, if your desire is to wake up out of the fog of thinking. After all, it is easy to daydream your way through a day of comfort, a day of winning and success, but try daydreaming your way through intense pain, serious illness or intense mental suffering and you will find it nearly impossible. You may still find yourself lost in thought, but if you are determined to wake up, you will discover that these unwanted guests can be a great help. And for now, they are here regardless, so will you use them to wake up, or to add more suffering to your life?

Day 7: Living Mindfully: Allow everything

Allow and Improve

This is what 'allowfulness' means: we just allow the fullness of this moment. We are not even accepting it; acceptance requires some effort. You have to try to accept, you have to work at it, and you have to come up with reasons to make it OK. Allowfulness, on the other hand, is just being here, curiously observing what is happening now – watching it and sitting with it. And in the curiosity and the watching, resistance disappears. But we don't try to change the resistance; we allow it to be there too. Instead of trying to accept, we allow the moment to be exactly as it is – no holding back, no fear. But if fear does arise, we allow that too.

This means that regardless of what comes up in your mindfulness practice, you are doing it right. You cannot do it wrong because whatever arises in the moment, as you are sitting, is what is. You cannot argue with what is; you cannot change what is. But, and here is the beauty of allowfulness, you can act to do whatever is possible to improve your life, to improve this world and to improve your health – and mindfulness is a part of that.

We allow this moment to be as it is because there is no way to change it. But that doesn't mean you can't do something to improve your situation or change things for the better. If you are sitting there and you notice that your house is on fire, you won't sit and mentally complain that your house shouldn't be on fire. You won't sit there and analyse how the fire might have started or wonder why life is so unfair. You won't sit there projecting a future where the whole house burns down and you can't escape. You will stand up and get out of the house. You will take action.

Often in moments of pure crisis when there is no time to think, we step out of our mental arguments, and we act in whatever way the moment requires. We act as best we can, and we continue to act. People do extraordinary things in those moments – things they would never have thought possible and could never have done if they had stopped to think about it. It would have seemed impossible, and they wouldn't have tried. There are thousands of stories about such remarkable actions.

Allowfulness doesn't mean being passive; it doesn't mean sitting still and waiting for things to work out. It means actively engaging with what we see as difficult, embracing it, jumping into it and then taking the best action we can to improve things.

Activity: Grist for the Mill

As you stop judging, your experiences – good, bad, or indifferent – lose their labels of wrong or stressful or scary. You come to a place where suddenly every experience you have becomes food for your practice, fuel for your mindfulness. Your experiences bring deeper peace to your mindfulness practice and your life, even if you don't feel peaceful in the midst of those experiences. Fear drops away, and stress largely dissipates as you learn to embrace difficulty and challenge – to embrace even anger, sadness or frustration.

When you do that, life starts to flow with joy, ease and lots of laughter. You can actually look forward to finding the places where you are still a bit stuck (although you're never really stuck, just lost in your mind at times).

Take a few minutes today to write a list of all the situations and circumstances in your life that you resist. Write down anything that you find yourself mentally complaining about, anything that should be different. Now cross out everything that isn't happening now, as you sit and write, cross out anything that can't be directly observed in this instant. Next cross out everything that is here now, but can't be changed, as much as you would like to change it. And finally, look at what is left (if anything) and write down what peaceful action you could take to improve that situation.

Over the coming days, notice each time the mind wants to complain about the things on that list that either don't affect you right now, or can't be altered at this time. Don't suppress those thoughts, just watch. As you observe these mind patterns, awareness increases a little and the power of thought to control you continues to dissipate.

Sitting with What Is

As you sit this week, know that whatever happens in your practice is what's happening in your practice. You can't argue with what is; or rather, you can argue all you like, but you can't win the argument. If the mind is busy and you keep getting distracted when you sit, that is what is. Allow it. Work with it. If you feel resistance to allowing what is, then simply allow resistance to be there. Notice how it feels in this moment to resist what is. As soon as you look at resistance, it becomes just another part of this present moment, something else to pay attention to.

If anger arises – or sadness, frustration, grief or happiness – allow the feeling to be there, and become curious about it. You can even stop calling it anger or sadness or grief. You can step out of labelling the experience. You can just be there sitting, not knowing, curious.

You can notice: 'Hmm, there is a sensation in my chest. It is hot and tingly, or it's heavy or cold. Hmm, that is really interesting. What happens when I pay attention to it? Oh, it gets stronger. Now it disappears. Now it comes back.' All of a sudden, that feeling stops being a problem and becomes a part of your experience instead. In that instant, there are no problems, only things happening in this wonderful Now.

I hope you have enjoyed this week of allowfulness, and that you have begun to experience the joy that arises when we allow the world to be as it is. As we continue this journey together, we will explore those sights that you do not see, the sounds that you do not hear and the silence and stillness that ordinarily goes unnoticed.

WEEK 3

Space and Things

If you look around, you will see that there are two types of phenomena in the world: space and things. At least, that is what we see from our human perspective. On a cellular, quantum physics level, there is actually stuff everywhere, and there is no space. But there's no stuff either, and space is everywhere. (Trying to grasp this is completely mind-bending.)

From our perspective, however, there is stuff and space, sound and silence, activity and stillness. Our good health and happiness depend on a balance between these things – between rest and activity, sound and silence, light and dark, space and things. And you don't need me to tell you that humans are way out of balance when it comes to these phenomena.

This week, I invite you to explore your inner and outer worlds and to allow these two dimensions to find a balance within you.

Sound, Activity and Things

Our minds are always drawn to objects. The mind is primarily interested in sound and activity. You can test this by looking around right now. Notice what your eyes are drawn to and what your mind pays attention to. It's probably things – the pictures on the walls, the trees, the people, the buildings, the clouds (or maybe the fingerprints on the wall if you have kids as I do). Your mind is drawn to all those things. (I say your mind because even though the eyes take the image and the brain processes it, it is the mind that is focusing on particular things.)

Now look around again, and notice that the most prevalent thing is probably empty space. What the mind doesn't notice, especially in a closed or crowded place, is that the volume of objects is very low compared with the volume of space. We usually see only the objects and not the space.

Take a moment to notice the space around you. Really take it in – look at that space. If you are in a place where you can see words or pictures, notice how much empty space is often found around and in those things. Pay attention to that background of emptiness.

If you can, go outside and look up at the sky, and notice all the space there is. Think for a moment about how much of this planet we actually inhabit and utilise. Bring your imagination out to the edges of the atmosphere and down to the core of the earth. Then realise that humans live on the top six inches most of the time. And yet it is all the parts we don't use, the places that seem useless, that allow those six inches to be useful.

This week, we will take a closer look at what you may have

thought was useless – silence, stillness and space. We will explore the world that is hidden in our perception and we will see how noticing that which is hidden can bring balance, health and happiness.

Day 1: The Space in You

The Busiest Place on Earth

The busiest realm of activity for most of us is thought. Our minds spend all day and some of the night trying to label, describe and understand a world that is infinitely complex. This is a big job and, of course, it is never complete, so the mind keeps working and thinking, thinking and working. Take your attention to the world of thought for a moment and watch what arises. Notice how busy that world can be. In the midst of noticing, watch for any gaps between thoughts and silent spaces in the mind. We'll come back to that in a moment.

Because of the way it operates, the mind naturally separates life into compartments and focuses on certain parts while ignoring others. We tend to focus on activity as being good: it keeps us busy, demonstrates our worth to the world and prevents labels like 'lazy' and 'aimless' from sticking. We could say that the world has conditioned us to value action, to value stuff and to seek sounds and sights, while ignoring the wonders of quiet time, stillness and silence.

But if the world seems noisy and busy, this is no more than a reflection of your internal experience. You may be lost in thought (which is usually busy), and that thought-based existence is quite naturally stressful. In fact, so much of our thought is concerned with what we don't have, what we need and what should be different that of course it is stressful! You are 100 per cent perfect in this moment, and believing anything different is bound to feel uncomfortable.

When you pay deliberate attention to stillness, silence and space, you will be amazed how quiet the world becomes, how much downtime you have, and how relaxed you are compared to the rest of the human world. It is not stillness itself, but the awareness of stillness and the appreciation of stillness that brings about this change.

Identity and Activity

What activities define you as a walking story? What do you tell people when you meet them to demonstrate that you are someone who engages in valuable, worthwhile effort in this world? For most humans, the busy work that they do day to day becomes the basis for much of their imagined personality. I say imagined not because you made it up, but because that personality is based on memories and future projections, neither of which are real. If you take note of the conversations that arise when people meet for the first time, 'What do you do?' comes pretty high on the list. (Personally I prefer the question 'How do you do?' and the answer 'With great care and attention'.)

Perhaps the reason why humans are uncomfortable with stillness is that we fear the loss of identity that we imagine would accompany the suspension of thought and the physical activities we like thinking about. Who would you be if you weren't doing something?

Activity: Who am I Now?

Today I invite you to spend 20 minutes doing absolutely nothing. Not meditating, not reading, not drinking tea. Just sitting in silence, doing nothing. Not thinking about the past or the future, not planning, organising or anticipating, just sitting.

As you attempt this, notice what the mind does. Notice how it feels in the body, and what thoughts arise. And watch what happens to your identity, your sense of self, when activity is taken away.

The identity that we derive from activity is not about the activity itself, it is about the story of me. The story of me has a beginning, a present moment and (hopefully) a happy ending. The activity is not important in itself, it is only important as a step towards the future. When you sit and simply be, you challenge this pattern and you bring the unconscious to the surface. Most people are so trapped in the pattern of doing, of stepping towards the future, that they never manage to stop and notice the pattern itself. If they could, it would begin to dissolve, because it is largely unsatisfactory, it doesn't lead to fulfilment and the future success is always just out of reach (if only you could get this or that). The future never comes.

You have a deeper identity, which is stillness itself, the awareness that is there even when thought isn't, and providing space in your life provides space for this awareness to shine through.

Day 2: Listening with Love

Thoughts and Relationships

When I talk to my friend Julie (not her real name), I can tell she doesn't hear me. I can tell because I have to repeat it three times before she gets it. I can tell because her answer doesn't match my question. And mostly I can tell because of the halfway look. You might have seen the halfway look yourself, and I am certain you have done it. The halfway look arises mid-sentence, when I have enough information about what I think you're going to say to switch off a little and think about my response. And Julie is a master at this.

Now I love Julie dearly, even in the midst of that look, because I can look at her from a place of stillness. From there, everyone is a dear friend, even if they're confused. But Julie doesn't love me. She seems to, but in reality she loves her story about me, and in the midst of the halfway look, she is deep in that story.

Of course, Julie is just like the rest of us humans, she is in a controlling relationship with thought. It keeps whispering to her, telling her what to do, how to feel, and Julie gets sucked in almost every time. Caught up in thought, we become self-obsessed, because at its root, every story is, in the end, the story of Me. When Julie thinks about what I am saying and smiles, she interprets it through her story, she thinks about what that means for her, and she re-evaluates what she thinks of me. None of this has anything to do with me, in fact it cuts off the present-moment connection that could occur between us as I speak. That speech is an expression of my energy, and if Julie could be still and listen, we could connect on a deeper level, but when I speak, she can't manage this. Luckily, when

Julie speaks, I can feel my breath as I listen, I can notice distracting thoughts and refocus on her, and until she finishes I can sit, look and smile. And so the connection is there. When Julie speaks, her personality is out front, jockeying for position, wanting to be noticed. If my personality does the same, there will be a competition, but I have played this game, and I much prefer to be nobody. So I listen, empty of a yapping self, eyes clear, breathing slow, and we talk and we laugh.

I know what Julie is doing for one reason: I used to do the same (and occasionally I still do). I grew up seeing friendships as a competition to be the funniest, the smartest, the best, and although I was pretty good at the game, it always felt a bit hollow, and there was always a hint of anxiety. Many people live their lives like this and never notice another way. They keep score, work hard and lose heart when others don't like them as much as they should. This way of relating keeps me focused on you, but deep down, it's all about Me.

The strange thing is that, once you stop caring about others, you can truly care. When you stop concerning yourself with what people might think, what they believe, how they feel and what they should do, only then is a true connection possible. Before that, there is too much control, too much scheming for anyone to truly meet another. It seems counter-intuitive, but now that I don't care about you, I love you, even though we may never have met.

It is curious to note that, when I think about you, I am really concerned for me, because all my thinking is about me, but when I just look, without seeking to influence you one bit, I truly love you. Try this with a friend in real life and you may be shocked to notice how little you knew about them before today.

Activity: Don't Care, Just Love

Picture a dear friend or relative in your mind and consider all the things you hope they will do and experience. Think about how you would like that person to see you, how they should treat you, and how they could demonstrate their love. When you watch these thoughts, who do they all lead back to? Whose interests are at the core of this process? Yours of course!

Picture that person once more, but stop caring in the conventional sense. Instead, picture them in intricate detail, picture their face if you can, remember their voice, their way of moving, their tone and expressions. Do this out of pure interest, with no aim but to know that person better, and as you remember, be still and breathe. When you look in this way, who is the object of focus?

Day 3: Emotions in Space

A Curious Paradox

If you pay close attention, you will notice that silence and sound actually exist at the same time. When sound arises, what is it arising in? What allows the sound to be separate – to stand out and be distinguished? The answer is silence. There is silence in the background. As I speak, there is silence all around me, and out of the silence, the words emerge. If there were no silence, everything would be white noise. No one would be able to distinguish my words; we wouldn't be able to distinguish sounds.

Another example is a blank canvas and some paint. (To get a more accurate picture, imagine the paint is like pavement chalk that washes away in the rain.) On the blank background of the canvas, you can paint something. On the blank background of this page, you are reading these words; they're arising out of empty space. There is text, but most of the page is white. That white is far more important than the text, because without it no one would be able to see the words.

In the same way, the space around you right now is what allows you to live and to use the things you have. A kitchen table and chairs are not much use if your house is full of sand up to the roof. It is space that allows us to make use of objects. Space is what allows us to grow. It allows things to arise, allows a tree to shoot up. Look at a tree and notice how much room there is around it – how much empty space – it's wonderful! Even in the jungle there is a massive amount of space.

When powerful emotions arise, it can feel a bit like being trapped in the jungle. There is not much daylight coming through, you feel uncomfortable and there are vines, creepers and endless vegetation cramping your space. Many people find themselves pushed around by emotions and thought at this point, doing what thought suggests to get rid of the emotion or being pushed into an action they would not do on another day. Feeling depressed or anxious, you may avoid a job interview, leading to a sense of failure and increased anxiety and depression. Feeling angry, you might attack someone, causing more drama in your relationships, more confusion inside and a growing anger. The emotion and the thoughts that accompany it become all pervading, and like those jungle creepers, they strangle the life force out of anything else that tries to grow. Within this experience, it can be hard to recognise anything outside of that emotion, such is its power in that instant.

When emotions arise within us, they are brilliant attention seekers, especially painful ones. Emotions grab us, drag our attention away and monopolise our focus as humans. As we explored last week, these emotions feed negative thinking, which leads to pain, confusion and even more focus on the emotions themselves. But even emotions, if you look, arise in space, and if we can recognise what exists around those emotions, they quickly lose their power to frighten us.

Activity: Emotions in Space

Find a feeling in your body now, from mild stress or boredom to guilt, sadness, whatever arises. Notice the size of the emotion and the size of you. Check how much of your body it takes up. Is it two per cent? Five per cent? Maybe twenty at the most? Now check what is there around the emotion, the space, the energy flow, the warmth, all those different phenomena. Be aware of that emotion as a part of the physical experience in this moment, without allowing it to become overwhelming. Sit for a few minutes and observe what happens when you pay attention to the space around that feeling, as well as the feeling itself.

It is sometimes useful to dive into emotions as we did last week. At other times it may be more helpful to put them in perspective, to notice what else is happening. You may find this particularly helpful if the emotion is overwhelming, takes up a large amount of your focus and energy or prevents you from doing what you would like to do on a day-to-day basis. Keeping these emotions in perspective is a wonderful way to appreciate those sensations, without overemphasising their importance.

Day 4: Working with Stillness

Constant Activity

The same thing happens with sound and activity. The mind is drawn to them, and so we keep filling our days with more activities and our lives with more sound. We turn the radio on as soon as we get into the car. We book appointments back to back all day. We fill up our weekends. We turn the TV on as soon as we get home or as soon as we sit down after dinner – or even while we're eating dinner.

Places of physical quiet are getting harder to find. (I say 'physical' quiet because, as you will learn this week, when you find the space that is inside you, the outside world will seem quieter and more spacious, even though it hasn't changed.)

Sitting still and doing nothing for a few minutes seems to be one of the most difficult things for humans. On the other hand, most animals spend a lot of time sleeping, resting or lying down. If you have a dog, or especially a cat, you'll notice that it's quite happy to spend long stretches of time doing very little. Animals prefer that. They would get stressed if they had to be continuously active. They need that balance to survive and to thrive. But we humans have become generally uncomfortable with silence and stillness. Even reading this book might be a way to fill up your day or your night. (That's OK – don't stop reading.)

Finding Space

I work at a job where a lot of people are stressed. They are running from appointment to appointment, and they are busy. But I seem to have all this time, even though I am doing the same job as others and getting my work done. People tell me the story that I am doing a good job. I tell myself the same story (maybe it's not true). And yet I have all this space.

Before I started to practise mindfulness, I never noticed this space. I used to do jobs that were not that stressful, such as delivering pizza and things of that ilk. Yet I seemed always to feel very busy – and quite stressed at times. Now those feelings have changed significantly, and I believe it's because I have developed an awareness of the space and silence inside.

Watching those around me at work, I am amazed how busy everyone seems to be. My friend Angela (not her real name) is a classic example. She comes in before me, she leaves after me, she never takes a lunch break and she is often running from one thing to the next. I suspect Angela thinks I am a little bit lazy, because I practise the balance of space and things, of silence and activity, so when I am active, I am focused, dynamic and fast-moving. Other times, not so much. When I am still, I read books, I contemplate how I could work smarter and I analyse our systems.

Why doesn't anyone else stop to figure out a better way to work, to understand what has an impact and what doesn't, to check that we're heading in the right direction? Two things stop them: future and object focus. Future, as you will know, is that imaginary concept in your mind that you're trying to get to faster, and the best way to feel like you are moving forward, towards that happy future, is to do things, tick items on your list and generally appear busy. This is incredibly satisfying to the mind, because things are getting accomplished. Are those things of any value? Are they improving your work, your life and the world around you? That doesn't matter, as long as the list is ticked.

Object focus means an obsession with things to the exclusion of all else. Moving through the day, Angela has as many opportunities to stop as I do, but her mind tells her to keep going, and stopping feels like halted progress. Without objects to play with (thoughts, tasks, activities) Angela is stuck with her thoughts and uncomfortable feelings. Unsure how to manage these, she smokes between coffees, she obsesses over menial tasks and she keeps an object in focus at all times.

Angela is actually about the best person I have worked alongside, but I can only wonder about the potential she possesses, if only she were comfortable to move slowly at times, to stop and be still. The energy she expresses would then have the power of stillness, the power of creativity, the vitality of life. This is true power.

Have you ever watched big cats hunting? They exemplify this principle. A cheetah must save as much energy as possible for the one piece of activity vital to its survival this week – the chase. And so it uses stillness, silence and inactivity for hours at a time, saving it all for a 20-second burst a few times per day.

Day 5: Allowing Inspiration

Enjoying the Unknown

As you learn to embrace space and to sit with not-knowing, you become free to enjoy possibility and creativity. You don't

Activity: Becoming a Cheetah

Today, I want you to take a risk by strategically doing nothing. Take three five-minute periods at work or at home in the morning, midday and afternoon to do nothing. Just sit, be still, breathe and allow your energy to recharge. And when I say do nothing, I mean nothing. No tea, coffee or smoking, no reading, no chatting, just sit and breathe.

After you spend this time in stillness, notice what happens to your work, your energy and your attention to detail. And ask yourself: did I miss anything by sitting still for a moment?

need to jump to the answers so quickly. You can sit in the curiosity and the wondering. This is where true inspiration comes from. This is where truly good ideas come from – where decisions that resonate with you come from – because you are allowing the time for things to germinate. You are not trying to make the plants grow before they are ready. You are watering and watching and allowing, following the next possibility and the next possibility.

This week, spend some time reflecting on any places in your life where impatience is creeping in and uncertainties or unknowns are making you uncomfortable. You will want to fill the discomfort with something, but try to dive in and embrace the unknown. Use the transition as a time to be still and enjoy some rest. There is no need to avoid activity, but you can play with what life is giving you right now and experiment with the wonders of embracing those pauses.

See it as an adventure. Although you don't know what

will happen, you can allow the adventure to unfold on its own timeline – because what arises out of the unknown will be infinitely more interesting, exciting and fun than whatever your mind could have come up with. If you can allow the space, your life will unfold as it is meant to.

Embracing the Gaps

As you go about your day, start to notice the gaps between activities – for instance, when you are waiting at the bank or the supermarket or at a red light. Also pay attention to the time between appointments or before you go to bed. Notice those times, and start to embrace them by tuning in to your inner peace, quiet and stillness.

Ordinarily, people aren't very happy when waiting in a queue or at a red light. But these are times to stop, reset and tune in to what's happening now. If we can embrace the gaps and enjoy them, our world will instantly be a better and more relaxing place. So this week when life forces you to slow down, just slow down.

On a bigger scale, life sometimes puts gaps between what we see as our natural development or the expected order of progression. Sometimes there are gaps between relationships or jobs, or gaps between things that we think should be consecutive. It is often very uncomfortable for human beings to sit in that place of potential – that uncertainty about what is going to arise or be created next.

You have probably heard the saying 'If you create space, then something new will arise.' Sometimes leaving an old relationship makes space for something new to come along. But in that gap in between, people often get tempted to go back to the old or to fill the space with something – anything. It's similar to automatically turning the TV on at night.

But it is important to realise that space is the place of creativity and infinite possibility. It is the blank page before you start to draw or write or paint. There is no need to fear the space if you can just sit with it – if you can make friends with those gaps between events or life stages.

When we stop trying to fill the emptiness and just allow the space, then the next stage can grow naturally. You may have noticed that when you try to fill the emptiness prematurely, things don't seem to work out. They often fail, or you can't quite make them happen. But when you give up and wait, sometimes an opportunity suddenly arises and everything falls into place – it all comes together.

If we can embrace the uncertainty and the not-knowing, change is no longer difficult. When you can wonder about what is going to happen next, instead of thinking you know what should happen and exactly how, then change becomes both peaceful and exciting.

It seems like a paradox, but the key to creativity is being able to move smoothly between these two worlds, of stillness and activity. Inspiration often comes out of inner stillness mixed with outer activity. When the body is doing something but the mind is clear and focused, then brilliance can arise. In this space, you are engaged with this instant, but you remain grounded in the silence at the core of yourself. And when you become the bridge between stillness and activity, it is impossible to know what brilliance will arise in your presence.

Day 6: Appreciating Stillness

Balancing Stillness and Activity

Like things and space, stillness and activity are two sides of the same coin – you can't have one without the other. In some ways, stillness is simply the absence of activity. But the stillness inside is much deeper than that. It is the possibility of activity. It is infinite possibility. What could be created out of that stillness?

Activity dominates the human world, and our health suffers because of it. We emphasise the quick result, the next thing and another tick off the list. This affects the way we treat the body – with fast food and quick calories – and the way the body is affected by the mind – with the stress of striving for the future.

Many people get sick when they start their holidays because the body drops the adrenaline-fuelled rush and can finally stop, then the effects of that pushing kick in. To have balanced, stable mental and physical health, we must learn to appreciate the other side of the coin, we must learn to stop.

Appreciating Stillness

When was the last time you appreciated a moment of stopping and doing nothing? Did you savour the wait to check out at the shop? The long queue at the bank? Or were you impatient and lost in thoughts about the next thing you needed to do? When your car broke down and you got to sit by the side of the road for hours listening to the wind, did you embrace that quiet, or were you too busy looking at your watch, waiting for the recovery vehicle?

We often blame life for our busyness, but if you look closely and take some ownership of what's happening, you will see that when opportunities for stillness arise, we usually resist them. We prefer to be in perpetual motion, constantly on the move. Sitting still arouses guilt, as there is always something else to do – but for what purpose? Is it more important to 'do' or to enjoy your life? Will you find fulfilment through another mindless activity or through returning your attention to your actual life, to this present moment? Instead of busyness, humanity must seek balance.

The mind develops strong preferences for activity, sound and stuff. After all, these are things that can be separated, analysed and thought about. Try thinking about silence and there is nothing to grab on to! But if we can stop getting caught in the tendency to separate life into parts and to prefer certain things, then we can allow the balance of silence and sound, activity and stillness, thought and no thought. Yes, that's right, I said no thought.

When a thought arises, try to watch it and notice what it is arising in. What is the background? What's around it? Again, for you to distinguish the thought, there has to be a background of stillness and silence. A thought arises in the silence, stays for a bit and then disappears. Where is it disappearing to? I don't know. But what is left is silence.

Being physically and mentally healthy is more than just avoiding illness, it is the harmonious balance of stillness and activity. And as you become familiar and comfortable with stillness, it begins to flow into even the active parts of your life. There can be inner stillness amid outer activity and vice versa, and so you can appear busy but be inwardly calm, just as you can be physically still while in inner turmoil.

How many activities each day require some movement but don't require thinking? When you walk, when you brush your teeth, when you pour yourself a drink, is there any need to be thinking? In those simple, everyday activities, we can experience great benefits by simply allowing the inner world to slow down, by dropping the urge to rush on to the next thing. Taking this one step, notice the stillness inside; even if the mind is active, feel the breeze, notice the breath and enjoy this step, grounded in the peace that is there even when you are engaged in activity.

Activity: Physical Stillness

Take a breath and drop your attention into your body. Feel the breath coming and going as you explore the body from the inside. Notice the activity of the in-breath and the stillness between breaths – that moment in which there is a pause. Sit still and notice the feeling of being physically still; sense the endless possibilities of this moment. What will arise out of this? What will this body do next? Sink into that stillness and enjoy the feeling it brings.

Spend ten minutes in this stillness and notice what it is like. How does the mind react to sitting still? What emotions arise in that nothingness – peace, boredom, guilt? And was the activity you could have done in that time more important, more fulfilling than a little rest?

Day 7: Living Mindfully: Space, stillness and peace

Noticing the Silence

Your practice for this week has been to tune in to your inner space and silence. It is not necessary to create that silence: it is there at your core. In that depth there is no noise. You don't need to create silence – you just need to notice it. Notice the space that is there even in the presence of noise.

Modern Western life is almost completely full of things, or so it appears. In reality, though, things are what we notice, what we are attuned to, and what we value. Silence is all around you, and stillness exists everywhere, but a mind cannot see them. They cannot be labelled, cannot be con-ceptualised, so thought has no interest in them. And as we

---

Activity: The Space Between Breaths

Take your attention inside now and notice the breath. Feel the breath coming and going, and notice its rhythm. It may seem as if you are breathing continuously, but there are pauses – there are gaps in the breath. As you breathe in and out, notice those moments of stillness between breaths.

Once again I invite you to feel the in-breath, feel the out-breath, and notice any pauses during the breathing cycle. In those pauses, pay close attention to how it feels to sit still between breaths – to be sitting there doing nothing for that instant. (Of course, we are not really doing nothing. The body is doing a whole lot of things to keep us alive.)

Let yourself sink into the stillness between breaths and really feel it. Then allow the stillness to disappear as the next breath arises. This is very important because our practice is about moving beyond preferences. We can't do that if we get stuck in disliking activity and wanting stillness to stay around for ever. As the stillness disappears, shift your attention straight to the breath. Really feel the breath and the gap between breaths.

You can also take a moment to listen to the sounds around you – to really listen. Watch for any silences between sounds. Notice the silence that is there after the sound disappears. You can play with this by tapping on a glass or ringing a bell, or using anything with a resonant sound that slowly fades. Create the sound, and then follow it as it disappears into silence and the sound waves change into something else. Notice the silence that exists after the sound. Notice the silence that the sound fades back into, just as chalk washes from a pavement.

Now notice the gaps between thoughts. Watch what happens after one thought disappears and before the next one arises. Fully experience that inner quiet, and then let it disappear as the next thought arises. When you sit in those gaps, you realise – maybe for the first time – that the whole world is silent. It is silence masquerading as sound. It is silence taking all these different forms and then fading back into itself.

become increasingly obsessed with things, people keep telling me that the world is speeding up, that the years are going faster, that everything is more complex.

But as I become untangled from the mind, I notice the opposite. The world I inhabit is slowing down. The planet I live on is becoming gradually simpler. And I have no idea what the date is, so how could the years go quickly?

To be invested in things is to be invested in the unreliable, the unstable, what the Buddha called 'impermanence'. This is a shaky foundation from which to seek peace, but the mind, which is no more than a recogniser and labeller of objects, is unable to see anything else. On the other hand, the still, silent awareness that is who you really are is immovable, unshakeable and dependable. Investing in this world of stillness is very sound.

And it seems clear that the biggest commodity you can invest is your attention, so where will you place it?

Attuned to silence, you escape from the stream of thinking. Connected with stillness, you stand firm in this world of change.

WEEK 4

Discovering Your True Self

Discovering your true self may sound deep and mystical, but the exercises and your practice this week will make it very concrete and real. You will actually experience your true self, rather than talking, thinking or philosophising about it.

If you have studied meditation or mindfulness, you will have learnt about all the things you are not. The Buddhist teachings are great for this, and mindfulness, too, teaches that you are not your thoughts, your feelings, your experiences, your job, your body or your name. All these things are changeable. In fact, I will start with the radical notion that anything that comes and goes – anything that changes due to external or internal conditions – isn't you.

From there we can explore what you really are if it is not these changing phenomena.

I want to forewarn you that some of the content this week is going to sound philosophical and theoretical. Your mind is going to want to argue with it and challenge it, to say, 'Yeah, but ...' and 'What about ...?' That's OK. I urge you not to get caught up in the words, but to do the exercises and check for yourself. Treat this as an experiment. I say you are not your thoughts, but don't believe me and don't disbelieve me. Experiment for yourself.

Day 1: Loving Who You (Really) Are

Looking at Identity

This week, your job is to look inside and see what you find. Incredibly, when we do this, it is very difficult to find anything solid. If you really look for yourself inside, there's nothing that you can grab on to. There's nothing that you can point to as being you.

The most prominent thing in most people's lives is thought, and it is from thought that we derive our identities: I think, I believe, I have this opinion, and on and on. But when there are no thoughts, who are you? And when your thoughts change, does that mean you are a different person? Of course, we often say that we are: I have changed; I think differently now; I am a different person from who I was then. But have you changed, or are you just having different thoughts?

Thoughts are merely part of your experience right now, like the wind and the waves and the person walking past, or the car horn honking or the birds singing. These are all part of your experience of this moment, and then they are gone. Thought is gone almost before you can catch it. Even when you're ruminating, and a pattern of thought is coming and going, coming and going, changing slightly, and coming and going, each individual thought is still arising quickly and then vanishing.

You may notice some thoughts drifting around, some

beliefs and some memories, but these are all coming and going, like the wind and the clouds and the dust. Of course, there is the body, but that keeps changing too. What we call our identity is a loose conglomeration that we don't want to look at too carefully because it's actually pretty unstable. Our body is unstable, and our thinking patterns and beliefs are unstable – they change all the time. Memories change. We lose memories, and we build memories that perhaps aren't quite accurate, according to others. All of the things that you call Me are ultimately unreliable.

Activity: Look Inside

Go inside and look for yourself, because maybe I'm right and maybe I'm wrong. Maybe I've missed something that you will find. See if you can find something that's you – something concrete that you can point to – something that's not changing, that won't be different in a week or a month or a year or 50 years. What will be left then? What will be the same?

Try not to consider this with the mind. Try to just look inside and wonder. Bring curiosity to the search. See whether you can find something inside that you can point to and say, 'That's me.'

Notice feelings, stress, sensations and the breath itself arising in the body, and ask yourself who is watching them. Who is feeling them? The nerves are sending signals to the brain, but who is there, watching and feeling?

When you sense yourself as the one who is watching, then take your mind back through your life and you may notice some interesting things. If you are like me, your whole body has changed even in the last ten years. It looks different, it behaves differently and it has different capabilities and different problems. (Actually, every cell has been replaced. Your whole body has died and regrown. Amazing, but true.)

Your thoughts are also different from what they were 10 years ago, or 20 or 30 years ago. Your beliefs have changed. Your life situation is different – your job, your friends, or your partner. There may be some constants, but a lot of things will have changed.

And everything about you and your life is different now from when you were a child. But there is one constant running through it all, and that's You. But it's not You the personality, or You the mind, or You the brain or the body – it's You the one who watches – the one who is watching right now. You are still here.

That You has been lost in thoughts. It has been walking through this mist and fog. And you have been thinking that you are the fog or the mist, when in fact, you are the one walking through it. That You has fallen asleep. It is in this dream world of story, which is a fine place to be, but it's not reliable. You're creating stress, anxiety or excitement in the body, but to You the watcher, none of it is real. You are having a dream. You're not really in the mist; you're caught up for a while in the world of story.

If you want to, you can wake up now – wake up out of thought. When you notice yourself as the one who is watching, you are waking up to awareness and to your true self.

And what if you could live your life from there? What if,

instead of remaining a small, confused speck in this large and complicated universe, you could get in touch with your true self, pure awareness? If you can, you will find that all fear disappears, because what does awareness have to fear? You will find that all bickering and competition ends, because you will realise that all others are pure awareness too. And you may find yourself drowning in peace, even when the external world seems wild and chaotic.

Notice what thoughts are passing through your mind right now; listen to them. You are watching them as you would watch a movie, and you are not the movie. Because you can watch your thoughts as they come and go, thoughts are not who you are.

Your thoughts are not who you are, and your beliefs are not who you are either. Your beliefs are mostly not even yours; they are a bundle of thoughts that you inherited and believed in – some repetitive stories that got stuck.

What Stays the Same

I've talked about all the things that keep changing, but there is something inside you that has stayed the same. You do have an identity of sorts. There is one constant in your life: the awareness that exists in the background, watching.

But when I say that your identity is awareness, don't believe that either. See what you find when you go inside and do the exercises. In fact, believing what people tell you – what you hear in classes or read in books – may be the biggest barrier to discovering yourself and waking up out of thought. Use what people tell you to spark your curiosity, and then verify things against your own experience. That is the key.

The Awareness that Watches

My experience is that when I look inside, I can sense myself. I can sense myself watching, but the me that I sense is not the personality, it's not the thoughts, it's not the beliefs and it's not the body – it is just consciousness, just awareness.

I can sense the fact that I'm aware and I know I'm here experiencing this life. I don't really know where I came from. My parents tell me a story about that, but I don't really know because I don't remember. I don't know where I was before that. I don't know where I'll be after this body dies. I don't know what happens next.

If I continue on this path, I'm almost not sure whether what I think has happened in my past is true. I know that my memory of what happened today is unreliable. It is a perspective. If all the people who experienced those things with me disappeared from the face of the earth, I would have no way of proving that those things happened. It would be like a hallucination. (And actually, this is not a disorientating feeling at all.)

Go inside now and notice what thoughts are passing through your mind. Watch them, and let them come and go. As they drift past, ask yourself who is watching the thoughts. Who is it? Who is aware of the mind? It's not the mind that is aware. The mind is just thinking and producing thoughts.

As you watch the thoughts, notice how they come out of nowhere. You don't control them. You don't get to choose what comes up or how long it stays. Thoughts just come, stay and vanish. Of course, you can try to control your thoughts, and you may be able to exert some control for a short amount of time. But it has been well documented that if I tell you not to think about bananas, you will soon be picturing a big yellow banana and imagining yourself peeling and tasting it. You won't be able to avoid thinking about bananas for long, no matter how hard you try.

So as thoughts arise and disappear on their own, just notice that there is someone watching. As you read, you can ask yourself, 'Who is looking at the words?' The eyes are doing something, and the brain is doing something, but who is taking it in? Who is making sense of it? The mind is saying things about it, but who is observing it in the first place?

Nothing to Change

This is where most meditation teachings and teachers lose their way, because they have been fooled by the mind into thinking that meditation is a way to train yourself – that it's a way to improve yourself or cultivate something in yourself. Nothing could be further from the truth. There is nothing that needs to be cultivated. There is nothing that needs to be changed.

All you need to do is to get in touch with your true nature. That is all we will practise this week. When you do that, everything else takes care of itself. But when you try to train yourself, your practice becomes an effort. It is difficult and challenging. And naturally, you set goals. You have future hopes, and you begin working towards something, which immediately and unavoidably takes you out of the present moment.

Day 2: Awareness of Emotions

Looking Inside

When emotions arise for humans, it is easy to see that we habitually identify with them. Like my friend Angie, who puts on the face that says she is fine, but whose body and behaviour tell a very different story. Angie is up and down the hallway like a gazelle, walk-running from meeting to meeting as she dips from half of this meeting to half of that, always running late, always apologising.

I used to think Angie just had a big job, but later I realised that whatever our driving inner force is, our life will reflect that back. And so people who feel anxious and tense may seem perpetually busy, regardless of how many things they have to do. And when Angie walk-runs off to the next meeting, I can almost sense the thoughts and emotions racing through her body and mind, pushing her on to that future she never quite gets to.

Sitting at the keyboard right now, I notice my mind egging me on too, tracking how many words to go and keeping score. It reminds of the date this book is due to the publisher, but the body doesn't respond. Focused on each breath, aware that I am the one watching the thoughts, not the thinker, all is peaceful and calm. Most of the time.

But sometimes I forget too, and I drift into that world of future fears, lost in daydreams of events that may not happen, in places I may never again visit, and then the anxiety starts. It's like a lump under my ribcage on the left, a solid block that, 15 years ago, would have driven me to open a can of something, go to the fridge or turn on the TV. Back then, I was just like Angie. I played basketball six times a week while working three jobs and going to nightclubs at the weekend. Why did I run from thing to thing like this? Because I was scared. Not scared of life, but scared of that lump under my ribcage. That almost seems funny now.

You see, the lump is still there at times, but the fear is gone, because that anxiety is something I am watching, not something that I am. It's just another part of life's rich tapestry. Without the fear, I can choose what I do and how I live this life. Governed by the fear, I was constantly running. Are you?

Activity: What Drives You?

Take a pen and a piece of paper and complete these sentences without thinking about your response. Write quickly without filtering and see what comes out.

I only (*insert behaviour*) because I don't want to feel (*describe sensation*).

If I could sit with (*insert emotion*) I would much rather (*insert alternative behaviour*).

When (*insert emotion*) arises, I notice it as a (*describe sensation*) in my (*describe where it arises*).

Write these sentences for as many commonly occurring emotions as you can.

This simple exercise can help shed some light on your emotional life. After all, if you recognise that emotion, when it arises, as a sensation, not as a problem to be attacked, you can be the watcher of the emotion, the witness of that energy arising. When you are the witness, it matters less what the emotion is, because you will feel at peace anyway. Your happiness is no longer tied to particular emotional experiences.

And here we discover the freedom that comes when you know who you really are. There is no longer any need to run away from any internal experience. Instead we can use these feelings as fuel for our mindfulness practice.

Challenges as Reminders

As you learnt in Week 2: Allowfulness, challenges can become blessings. They can point you back inside again and again. Once you are there, those challenges will begin to disappear, because you won't need them to point you back inside any more. You will be inside – as just awareness – and it won't matter what the external world does.

Challenging emotions can become powerful reminders that you are lost in thought. In that instant of noticing those feelings, you can check who is watching and return to this place of simple, open awareness. There is nothing to achieve, no emotion to get rid of, just you watching an experience arise and disappear.

When you realise that there is no need to do anything about those feelings, you can keep coming back to awareness again and again, reminding yourself over and over to return to this instant. And when you drop out of that awareness, you just come back to it again. As you spend more time living this awareness, it starts to strengthen, and other mind patterns dissipate.

That is all this practice is. There is no training and no cultivation. You don't need to change anything about yourself. Everything that happens in your life and in your practice is nature's way of pointing you back inside. Whether things go right or things go wrong, they are pushing you to look at that inner world. So, whenever you feel challenged, remember to feel what is happening in your body, rather than thinking about it. Connecting with the body like this, your attention is centred once more.

Make emotions your friends and your practice will grow strong, and you will know who you really are.

Day 3: True Relationship

No Differences

What if you could relate to others from your deepest nature, with no need to compare conditioning or act out the crazy mixed-up self we become when the mind is in control? Imagine if when you looked at another person, you just saw yourself, looking back at you, nothing more, nothing less. This is possible.

When I meet new people, I fall in love very quickly, but not in a weird way. I fall in love with them because when I look into their eyes I see me, pure awareness, hiding under a bunch of thoughts, concepts and behaviours. It's always fun to meet yourself.

It's a bit like the relief I felt travelling overseas when I met someone who spoke my language, who was Australian even, who would get me. After being surrounded by lovely people I couldn't connect with due to language or culture, I believed I had found someone with whom I could bond, because we were the same.

Years later, and with less thinking in the way, I see this everywhere, as every human, every animal has that same open awareness behind their eyes.

I think that's why babies are so similar when they are newborn. They have slightly different temperaments and characteristics, and obviously, they had different experiences in utero, so babies have some variation in temperament and other attributes at birth. But newborn babies are generally very similar. Over time, their conditioning grows. If you look at one-year-olds, there are some differences, but they're still reasonably similar. But if you meet two people at age 70, they have a lot of conditioning. It is really thick and hard to penetrate. But still, underneath that, they are the same.

If we picture identity (who you are at your core) and conditioning (what you think and believe based on your unique life experiences) as different, this sameness makes more sense. Every human is unique in terms of their physical form and their conditioning, and every human is the same at their core. When you realise this as you look into the eyes of another person, a barrier that seemed so real may melt away. No matter what people say or do or how they look, underneath all that conditioning, they are the same as you. There is no difference between any of us. We are in different bodies, we are living different lives and we are having different experiences, but all that will end. And outside of those things, there is no difference between us whatsoever.

Back in the ordinary mind, every other person is turned into a mental object that is liked or disliked, is good or bad, and (most important) is better than or not as good as me! This process separates us from our shared humanity, it leaves us feeling like small, vulnerable parts in an enormous, moving world and, most damaging of all, it allows a layer of mental noise to separate us from every other human, even if we say we love them. I love you, not because you can do something for me or because you're a good person, but because love flows naturally when I remember who I am.

Activity: Your True Identity

Take a minute now to watch thoughts coming and going. You may find it helpful to feel yourself breathing in and out. Feel the breath coming and going in the lungs. And as you do, watch what thoughts drift past. Notice all the different phenomena – the breath, the thoughts, the sensations – and notice yourself watching it all. You are there in the background as the watcher. You are there feeling excited, or you are there feeling peaceful. You are just there observing, letting everything come and go.

Whenever you get lost in a thought, come back to the breath and notice who is watching. Who is watching the breath? Who is watching the thought? Stay with that awareness as long as you can. When you get lost, just go back to it.

And as you walk around the world today, see if you can look upon someone else, another human, from that

> pure awareness. Look without concern for what your mind
> says about them or about the world, look for the sake of
> looking, and notice yourself there, watching at the same
> time. As you do so, you may sense that, underneath all
> that extra stuff, you are looking directly at yourself. How
> cool is that?

If this is the only practice you ever do, and if you keep doing it, you will realise your true self. You will find that you are more peaceful and happy than you could have imagined. It is that simple. There is nothing you need to do or to become. All you need is to realise who you are.

Day 4: Work without Ownership

Using Your Mind

Working without a strong sense of self – based on thought – may sound a bit strange. I mean, if you don't play the role of somebody, then won't you stop caring about completing tasks or achieving goals? Isn't it that sense of personal achievement that drives us as humans and allows us to accomplish great things? Well, yes and no. It is true that having an analytical mind is a great asset when you want to create new things in this world, and it is also true that you can use your analytical mind without it using you. What I mean is that, for most people, the mind tells them what to do. They react to thoughts and attempt to achieve things because they are driven by that mental noise.

Imagine you want to raise a new idea at work, something revolutionary that could significantly improve things for your team and those you serve. Even raising the idea in a team meeting may feel stressful because the mind takes ownership, seeing it as *my idea*, which in turn becomes *my possible failure*. If the team rejects it, or if the plan fails, it is my failure, something that feels threatening to the mind. But what if you could let go of that possible future outcome and focus instead on what is here now: a new idea. You could raise that idea and evaluate it with your colleagues, using the insights of others to build on or adapt it, while being prepared to let it go if necessary. This process would proceed with a sense of inner peace, curiosity and calm, leading to less resistance from others, more flexibility within your team and a sense of true collaboration. Whether this team is your work team, your family or your friends, this approach works. I know because I use it.

Without the need to achieve in order to make me seem special, I can still create. In fact, I create better work and am regularly struck by good ideas because I have an analytical mind, but am calm, clear and present. Great ideas can only arise when your mind is clear, because a repetitive stream of thinking won't let anything new arise.

It's fair to say that once I believed I was *this* person of *this* age doing *this* job, whereas now I know I am playing the role of this person. And playing that role is a lot more fun.

Playing a Role

You can still play the role of this separate person and enjoy it; I certainly do. And I also get lost in that role at times. When I do, life feels different; I get frustrated, stressed and annoyed –

or anxious and excited about the future. But even in the midst of that I always know deep down that when I step out of all that, when I wake up again, there is no concrete reality to it. It is just a role.

In the workplace, most people identify with their role, saying 'I am the senior manager' or 'I am a cleaner', and the identification with these roles, the ownership of them, causes stress. Success or failure starts to seem very important if it threatens your sense of self, and this leads to an interesting paradox. People who are overly anxious about keeping their role and protecting that part of their identity rarely do great work, and are therefore more expendable in the modern workplace.

Activity: Having No Future

Take a moment to imagine how your life would be if the future didn't matter. Of course, your mind is going to say, 'Well, if the future didn't matter, I wouldn't do anything. I would sit around and watch TV.' But maybe, just maybe that isn't true. Let's find out ...

As you sit there, reading this, see what it is like to make this instant your only focus. Forget about any future plans and past memories, just sit and take care of what you have to do right now. If something is on your to-do list, but you aren't doing it now, forget it. If something happened yesterday, let it stay in the imagined past. Act as if there is nothing to do, nothing to achieve, except what you are doing this instant.

Sit in that nowness for a few minutes and notice what it's like.

Those who have no concern for their future, but focus exclusively on doing brilliant work today often achieve great things and are very hard to replace. It seems that the more you worry about the future, the worse it will be, whereas the more you drop the future, the more success you will enjoy.

It is a common myth that it is the focus on the future that drives progress and achievement, but the hidden truth is that all great things are achieved with painstaking attention to the details of this instant. And when you live life from this place you will be surprised to find that results take care of themselves.

The actuality is that having no future will give you a lot more energy and a lot more drive to go out and enjoy Now. Surprisingly, you can still work towards future goals. It doesn't matter whether you reach them or not. You can still make plans, and you can still be organised. You can still do all those things, but the outcome will not be a source of stress for you.

The Death of Problems

Think about everything you have worried about this week, and then ask yourself how much it will matter in 20 years. How much will those things matter in a hundred years? There are very few things that will even be remembered in a hundred years.

What problems did your great-great-grandparents have that you know about today? I don't know of any. Of course, we know about historical events like the Great Depression or World Wars I and II, but what of the disagreements, family arguments and day-to-day worries? My guess is that they have faded into oblivion.

Perhaps they worried about how they would get another job, how they'd pay for X or what would happen if Johnny didn't go back to school. And yet none of those things are still important today – none of them.

Your problems will be dead in a hundred years, easy. And a hundred years is nothing. Dinosaurs died out 65 million years ago, and they were around for 180 million years. (I know this because I live with a five-year-old.) Actually, most of our problems will be dead in ten years – it's just that our minds will tell us we have new ones.

When you work this week, hold those so-called problems lightly. See them as opportunities to be present, challenges that can bring forth great awareness. And try to make the act of living this instant more important than the imagined outcome for an imagined you. Live as if you don't exist outside of this instant, as if the story of you was no more than a reference point, a way to make sense of the world around you. Allow it to do that, and no more, and see what happens next. You may be surprised to discover that your best work comes out of pure awareness, that it's not your work at all.

Day 5: No Self, No Worries (Free to Be)

Creativity and the End of Stress

My friend Helen is a worrier. She talks non-stop (amid a few laughs) about the stresses of her world whenever we meet for lunch. She complains about what should be, concerns herself with what might be and laments what was but is no longer. Helen is stuck in her head. Lucky for me (and Helen), she is also incredibly funny, and in the middle of all the woes, there is a shining humour about the underlying joke of it all, but still, Helen is lost in thought.

But when Helen picks up a crayon, a piece of chalk or a paintbrush, something magical happens. She loses all that worry, the unfairness seems to disappear and, all of a sudden, she is lost in her art. And her art is incredible. Of course, Helen won't admit this, because when she finds her 'self' again (the complaining one, that is), then it evaluates the work it was absent for and complains about that too. That thinking mind is a scared little critter, and it needs to reassert itself. But, sitting and watching, I know that there is more to Helen than that voice of complaint.

Creativity, as it turns out, is who you are, not a quality you possess, which is why Julia Cameron, author of *The Artist's Way* insists that we are all creative, though some may be blocked. But it would be more accurate to say that everyone is creativity rather than saying we are creative, because the very energy that you are is the energy of the creative universe.

I know what you might be thinking: Oli is going all Zen-hippy on us, but think about it for a minute. Your body was created out of energy, sperm and egg, that combined to make something completely new and unique, something that never was before nor will be again, a complete study in uniqueness. And you too have created things that never existed, be they thoughts, sounds, pictures, salads or anything you have contributed to; each is a creation in and of itself. Your body creates blood cells, skin cells, energy; your mind creates desires, memories and ideas; the creative pulse of the universe flows through you, is you.

This Wild Ride

If you allow it, this energy can come into the world through you, whether you are artistically gifted or not. The power to create belongs to us all, but the mind will do what it can to block this wild ride. After all, allowing the universe to create through you necessitates a loss of control, a reduced sense of ownership and a diminished personal sense of self. It means we must give up our painful self-image, our limiting story.

Activity: Giving Up the Story

Realising all this may leave you in a place of fear, as your identity becomes a little more fluid. We don't know exactly who we are when that story-based identity starts to loosen up a bit, so it is normal to feel afraid at this point. Your identity is a story you have leaned on your whole life, and whether it is an identity you like or not, it still gives you some sense of stability, some sense of predictability.

But, for a moment, embrace this nobodiness and see what arises. Take a pen and paper and breathe and focus. Sense yourself watching, observing the events of this moment, and let the pen guide itself however it sees fit. Don't judge what comes out, just do.

And as this doing emerges, notice that you don't know what will come next. Watch as something new arises unexpectedly, without thoughtful planning or careful analysis, a new creation that will never arise again. Take note of the energy that flows with this process, and allow it to recharge you, this energy of creativity. Play in this energy for as long as you wish.

Ordinarily, you know who you are and what you do, and this blocks newness from arising. When that familiar story is taken away, or even loosened for a moment, the mind may become fearful. If you are feeling some fear now, or if fear arises this week, it's a good sign. Try to jump into it and experience it, knowing that fear is not you either.

Human Consciousness

As humans, we have this extra layer of consciousness that nothing else on the planet seems to have. But the energy we're made up of is the same as everything else. Quantum physicists have proved that the whole universe is made of the same stuff. It takes on different patterns and different arrangements, but the base of everything is the same. It is an energy that they can't pinpoint. (I love the fact that our best and brightest can't find it.)

Once you realise you are a part of this universal energy and awareness, the fear of not having an identity drops away. You have an identity – it's just not a separate identity. Of course, you still get to play with your separate identity for this lifetime, but you know it's not real. It's not true, and it's not all that important. Things that aren't real or important are a lot more fun. You can enjoy them much more than things that are real and important and serious.

And this freedom from your thought-derived self has a side benefit: it leaves you free to let creation come into this world through you. New things can arise, energy can flow and you make this world a richer place. That's how powerful you are.

Day 6: Freedom from Illness

The Pain that isn't Mine

Knowing who you really are has another interesting side effect when it comes to dealing with illness and injury, an effect that surprised me when I first noticed it. I was sitting nursing a sprained, swollen and bruised ankle after a game of basketball. I have played since I was seven (which is quite a while) so I had experienced this type of injury many times before, though not for a few years. In those olden times, when I was struck with such an injury I would mentally complain, I would worry about missing games and having permanent damage and I would feel like I was pushing towards this better future, the one in which I was healed. I didn't realise it at the time, but all that thinking caused extra stress that was completely unnecessary. It had no benefits and made the experience of being injured much more difficult. I never realised this because I didn't know that the thinking was causing that stress. I thought the event was causing it, or the pain or the inability to play or walk. I never questioned this because it was what I always believed: that life is what causes your worry or your happiness.

But this later injury was different. After years of mindfulness practice, I found something very interesting happening: I was no longer fighting with the situation. I almost enjoyed having a good excuse to sit on the couch with an ice pack. I felt delighted at walking incredibly slowly around town as it allowed me to really look at and listen to the world around me. And although there was pain and limitation, I remained more present, more alert and more peaceful throughout this time. The experience was completely different.

What was the difference? Why did that shift in attention cause such dramatic change? In the earlier injuries, the situation was my problem, a part of my story that should have been different, and my job was therefore to think my way out of it. In the later example, my sense of self had changed. I was no longer so caught up in the belief that this body is me, that these thoughts are me, so I was more able to experience this instant from the viewpoint of awareness. And that made an enormous difference.

Activity: Peaceful Suffering

This may sound contradictory, but it is possible to suffer physically without torturing yourself mentally, to feel pain and experience limitation in peace.

Take a moment to notice your breath right now and to observe yourself as the watcher of breath, the underlying awareness. Notice any aches, pains or less than ideal physical conditions, and breathe. Check for a moment whether they are your conditions, or whether they are simply one part of your experience of this instant. And remember, if you can see it, it's not you!

The next time you experience a physical limitation, from illness to injury to simple fatigue, see if you can simply notice it. Try to observe that experience deeply and without resistance. If the mind wants to tell stories and complain, then let it, but keep coming back to the experience itself. As you watch, keep sensing yourself as the awareness, as the watcher, and breathe. Continue for as long as you would like.

Once the illness ceases to be a problem that you own and must solve, you can enjoy taking good care of this body without worrying about how it fares. You can embrace the opportunities that the situation brings you now, rather than focusing on what you could be doing if only the world would obey your commands. And whatever happens, you can be at peace, which is an amazing gift.

It is interesting to note that what we were taught from birth is not true: the world does not cause suffering, it merely creates limitations against which the mind rebels. The rebellion is the cause of that suffering.

Now, ending the rebellion does not mean giving up on the body, or sitting quietly waiting for your ills to cure themselves. As you will note, I was on the couch with an ice pack (well into the night), and you may also need to take some action to help your body heal. But once this action arises out of a calm allowfulness of this instant, you can take action without polluting your body with stress. Calm and alert, you may discover a cure or treatment you did not know about, or you may live with what is unflappable peace.

Some illnesses are so serious that even suggesting this may seem inappropriate, but consideration of the worst-case scenario shows the power of this approach.

Imagine you have terminal cancer, with only six months to live, according to medical advice. You have tried every treatment you can find without success. Short of a miracle, your life will end very soon. If you knew that you had six months left of this life, how would you choose to live them? Would you wish to spend those months complaining, arguing with life and feeling angry about your situation? Or would you choose peace if you could? Would you leave this world content and deeply aware, even in the midst of physical suffering?

It is impossible to change what is. The only option is to fight it or embrace it. And when illness and physical decay strike (as they will for us all), which will you choose?

Day 7: Living Mindfully: Stop training and wake up!

No More Training!

When we try to train ourselves and to strive towards something, we lose the present moment, and we lose the practice. We also start to tie ourselves in knots. When I first started practising, I would set goals, such as, 'Within three weeks, I am going to be able to stay present for five minutes at a time.' Of course, when I was sitting, I was focused on working towards this future goal, which took me away from enjoying the practice in the moment. Therefore, I was absent.

Once I was absent, the mind would come in and start telling me that I was a bad practitioner and that my meditation was pointless – that I might as well give up and spend my time doing something else, because it wasn't working. It was a waste of time.

This caused me to struggle with my practice, until I discovered that the only thing I needed to do was turn inward – that we are all in the process of waking up. We are all waking up out of thought. Some people are very lost in thought, and some people are very awake, but we are all somewhere on that continuum.

Waking Up

The process of waking up from thought is similar to waking up in the morning. You will awaken eventually, but there are things you can do to help wake yourself up sooner and to stay awake. In the morning, if you get out of bed straight away when you first wake up, then you won't fall back to sleep. If you put your alarm on the other side of the room, you will have to get up instead of going back to sleep. If you open the curtains, your body will start to pump endorphins in response to the daylight, and you will get a little rush of chemicals to keep you awake.

As you do these things, you don't say, 'I'm cultivating awakeness' or 'I'm trying to get to a state of awakeness.' You just say, 'I'm getting out of bed, and this is how I wake myself up.' It is similar with meditation: you are not trying to gain any special qualities or wisdom; you are just waking yourself up.

It may seem as though you have new wisdom, because when you stop getting lost in thinking, then things become really clear. But it's not that you didn't know those things before; it's just that you were lost in the fog. You haven't learnt something new – some great new knowledge or information that you can show off – you have taken something out of the way. Staring at the thoughts kept you from seeing what else was there. Getting bamboozled by thinking made things difficult.

So there is a change, but we haven't created anything new. We haven't absorbed something from the outside that will make us better people – although that is what we have been trying to do our whole lives, isn't it? That is why the self-help market has boomed. A lot of us are looking for a quick fix, for an expert from outside to come in and tell us how to fix ourselves: how to fix our personalities, our relationships, our bodies or our finances.

But if we live by our hearts, if we live with a connection to ourselves, then we know what to do and when to do it. Of course, there are times when we need expert advice, and we can still get help from others, but we know they can't fix us. We know there is nothing to fix.

And so this process is more like evolution than change. You are becoming something new: a human who doesn't compulsively need to think.

The Problem with Cultivation

It's very important that you drop the idea of trying to cultivate something or trying to become something through your meditation practice, especially trying to become someone else. If you are trying to become the Buddha or the Dalai Lama or another person you admire, two things are happening. First, you are looking outside yourself for wisdom, which implies that you don't have it inside. Second, you are aiming to become something different in the future, which of course means that you are not good enough as you are now. As a result, you have stepped out of this instant and into trying to improve yourself.

It's easy to get caught up in that type of thinking because the mind looks for wisdom outside itself, and it seeks to become something better in the future. Those are the usual patterns of the mind. But if you want to practise mindfulness, you need to go back inside and look to yourself each time this happens.

Your Only Job

With mindfulness, your only job is to go inside, and go inside, and go inside again – to keep stepping out of the search for something external that is going to make you happy, including the externals of wisdom, religion and even spirituality. All of these things are useful for pointing you back to yourself and telling you to look inside, but they are not going to give you anything more helpful than that.

What I know is that when I go inside, underneath all of the conditioning and all of the thought and belief, what I sense is an awareness – the same awareness that is in you – the same awareness that is you.

Activity: Giving Everything Away

Try something radical today: give away everything you have. OK, wait, don't start packing, because every 'thing' that you have exists in your mind. Everything in your world exists as a mental image – that's the only way you can know it. Even sense perceptions – things you can touch, see and hear – only have reality through thought. The vacuum cleaner, the table, the window – without a thought, they have no name, there is only this.

Sit still for a few minutes and let go of every label, every belief, every thought that arises now. Give it away and see what remains. Sit and examine your internal experience and don't allow anything that isn't you to take attention. Give all that extra stuff away.

What is left?

This aspect of mindfulness may take some time to understand through your own experience, or it may take a second reading. It is worth noting that awareness is not something you can understand through logical, conceptual thinking, so if your mind is trying to grasp it intellectually, it won't be possible. Stay with the experience, keep looking inside yourself and you will eventually discover that which I cannot describe: the awareness that is you.

WEEK 5

Dropping All Barriers

So far, we have covered focusing our attention, shifting our perspective, noticing space and looking inside. This week we will examine the barriers to waking up, so that we can drop them. Those barriers come in four parts: expectation, control, thinking and identity. We will look at them in detail this week, exploring how we get tangled in them, what the costs are and how we can move beyond all barriers.

How to Drop Things

First, it is worth answering the question: what does it mean to 'drop' things? When we think of dropping something, it usually implies an active effort: we have to get rid of, throw away or change whatever we are holding on to. But this week you won't need to actively try to eliminate or change anything. In fact, doing so would only suck you into a battle with your thoughts again.

The normal way to drop something is to change old thoughts into new ones. But if we merely try to change our opinions, beliefs or feelings, we are going to get lost in thinking. We will be back in the same old cycle of believing something needs to change and trying to fix it for the future – meanwhile missing out on this wonderful present moment.

When I talk about dropping something, what I mean is replacing it – making a shift in attention. In other words, all you need to do is pick something else up. For example, to drop a thought and stop playing with it, shift your attention to the breath. If you do that really intently, and you keep coming back and coming back, then the thought 'drops you', as Byron Katie says. You don't need to actively get rid of the thought; you can simply change your point of focus, shift your awareness. The way to drop something is by paying attention to and embracing something else. This will take you beyond all the barriers.

Imagine holding two hot potatoes, wrapped in foil, one in each hand. If you feel the pain in your hands but don't realise it is caused by the heat in those potatoes, you might go along thinking pain was part of life, unavoidable. But what if you swapped one of those hot potatoes for a cold one? You would feel a wave of relief in one hand as the pain reduced, and you would quickly realise the source of the problem. That realisation would lead to the end of your pain as you would drop the hot potato immediately.

Our practice this week will be similar. I will invite you to experience the opposite of the usual, painful way of living, and in that experience you will notice how much more enjoyable it is to live in the now. Therefore we need not make the mind into some sort of problem to be solved or got rid of; we can experience life without thinking and let the rest take care of itself. It's not quite as simple as the hot potato, because we are addicted to thinking, and even noticing the pain caused by an addiction won't necessarily stop it immediately. There is some detox to do, a withdrawal process and a transition from the life we were used to and were comfortable in, to a life of fulfilment. And rather than the 12 steps often used to move beyond addictions, we remain always at Step 1: be here now.

Day 1: Dropping Your Small, Painful Self

Dropping Identity

The first thing we will drop this week is identity. This can be the scariest of all, but fortunately, you have already done it. That's because when you drop thinking, you drop identity too. Identity is only there when you are thinking yourself into existence.

This doesn't mean that thinking keeps you alive physically, or that you will lose your mind if you learn not to think. But everything that you call Me is based on a thought. For example, your identity doesn't come from your body's characteristics – it comes from the thought that your body is fat, thin, ugly, pretty and so on.

Likewise, it's not that your job is who you are, it's that what you do makes up the content of a lot of your thoughts. The thoughts are saying, 'I do this and I do that, and what about this person? What does that mean? They should be more, or I should be more, or I should get more ...'

Even your family and your past aren't your identity. They are just what you think about and what your mind is concerned with. The mind is continually replaying memories of the past – the stories and movies and sound bites. But it's all just the content of your thoughts.

Activity: Who Owns That Thought?

I am making an assumption that most of the thinking you do is centred around the story of your life, the experiences and future of the person you believe yourself to be. Let's check that assumption before we go any further, in case your experience is a different one.

For the next few minutes, make thought the focus of your attention, but instead of thinking, simply watch each thought come and go. Treat thoughts like birds flying past outside your window, letting them come and go in their own time without engaging with them, chasing them away or trying to change them in any way.

As you watch, notice the themes that arise in those thoughts. When are they about: the past, the future or now? Who does the content of those thoughts relate to: you or others? And if they relate to others, are they primarily about how others treat you and how their behaviour makes you feel, or are those thoughts genuinely concerned with others?

Take a few minutes to get a better understanding of the thoughts that happen to you. It may be helpful to use breath awareness to anchor yourself in that place of watching, as the thoughts will try hard to pull you out of mindfulness and into thinking.

Finally, notice who is thinking. Is it you? Or do the thoughts just appear? If they appear without your control, who owns those thoughts?

Of course, many thoughts may seem altruistic and compassionate, but often what they are actually concerned with is what I want. Sometimes what I want is world peace, or for you to be happy, but it's still for my sake, because then I will feel better.

All these thoughts are important because they make up my identity, they tell me who I am. This is the source of the addiction, because without those thoughts, who would I be?

When thinking drops, identity drops with it, even though thought may still be there. I invite you to continue practising not-thinking by watching thought. You don't need to do anything else. You don't need to try to have different thoughts, just watch. Sometimes people get caught up in trying to create different beliefs, such as, 'I have no identity. I was never born. I am the original ...' and that kind of thing. This creates another barrier between you and the experience of you – another barrier to experiencing yourself.

Dropping the Burden of Me

When you shift from thinking to watching, you realise for the first time that identity was a burden – that it was actually something heavy getting in your way. Even if you have good self-esteem, maintaining your identity is a lot of work. You feel worried and anxious when that identity is threatened physically, or more often, psychologically; for instance, when someone criticises you, isn't nice to you or doesn't like you.

These psychological threats leave us fearful or angry, but if we are not trying to protect an identity, we can experience the situation and be done with it. Either there is nothing we need to do, or there is some action that feels right and we act.

Most often, the everyday dramas that people get into with other people lose their importance. We can let other people take care of their business, and we can take care of ours. As a result, life becomes incredibly straightforward and simple. Of course, you still get to keep your worldly identity. But you don't need to worry about maintaining or protecting it. You can live day by day instead.

Today, you have the rare chance to live not as a little me, but as a moment-to-moment expression of life. As you begin this process, you might feel disoriented, you may feel withdrawals, and you may start to notice how much energy is wasted in pointless thinking. As we continue this week's journey, remember that at any time you can move from thinking to living, simply by feeling yourself breathe.

Day 2: Dropping Resistance and Letting Emotions Flow

Releasing the Power of Emotion

Stress is tiring, and when I look at Frank, I can see it in his eyes. His body too shows the signs of blocked emotion – the rounded shoulder, the slight lean forward and the furrowed brow that has spent too long thinking about what might be. Frank's energy seems blocked, not because of life or even lifestyle, but because he is at war with his inner state.

When Frank feels that stress, if he knew how, he would use it to return to body and breath, he would come back to now. But because Frank thinks that life is causing his stress, he keeps trying to think his way out of it. This thinking is an attempt to escape from the physical sensations that we call emotions, and Frank doesn't realise that the thinking actually strengthens and reinforces those emotions instead of removing them. And so Frank is lost in this cycle, completely unaware that his way of living is the source of all his suffering.

Perhaps you can relate to Frank's way of being – I know I can. For more than two decades I lived the same cycle, convinced that if I could figure life out by thinking about it enough, I could find peace. Looking back I can see that the peace I sought was simply the absence of the emotional experiences of which I was frightened. I didn't want to live with the worry, the anxiety or the anger, and, thinking that life was the cause of these emotions, I put all my energy into two activities: figuring it out (thinking about life) and distracting myself (avoiding emotions).

I was lucky that I don't do things by halves, so when I used alcohol as a distraction for a few years, I did it very thoroughly, to the point that it was starting to have an impact on my relationships and my quality of life. And in the midst of this, I realised that, as well as causing harm, it wasn't working; the emotions were still there.

When I decided to stop drinking, I got hooked on TV. When we got rid of our TV, there was just me and my emotions, and I discovered something surprising. When I curiously explored an emotion in my body, the first part was hard, scary and painful. As I became more comfortable with that sensation, I noticed that it seemed to start to move. It went from a static, stuck sensation to a dynamic ball of energy. I realised that these sensations are no more than trapped energy, an interruption of the flow of life, and that if I allowed it to, that energy could become a flowing part of my life force.

Activity: Letting Emotions Flow

Take a moment to scan your body now for any stuck emotions or any aches and pains. As you tune in to the inner experience of the body, allow the sensations of the breath to anchor your attention in this instant. Bring a friendly attitude to those emotions or aches, smile at them as you would a scared child in a shopping centre, and let the breath flow.

As you sit still, watch for any movement in those sensations. See if they are static or if they are vibrating, moving or changing shape. Be attentive without forcing your opinion of what they should be doing on to these sensations. Allow them to be. Know that they will move on when they are ready, and be prepared to sit for eternity (which is only this instant after all) as the friendly, smiling watcher of these energy forms. Spend a few minutes allowing the flow of breath and smiling at your new friends.

The flow of energy is essential to the health of any system. The flow of ideas, discussion and banter makes for a healthy workplace; the flow of rivers and the movement of air currents promotes health in an environment and the flow of breath, the transition of water and food and the physical movement of the body lead to physical health. Emotional health is no different – it relies on the free flow of emotional energy, without which you will become stagnant or repressed. That energy wants to move, and you may find yourself exploding as anger moves, crying as sadness moves or fretting as waves of anxiety flow through your body. But with this simple skill, of sitting, watching and allowing that flow, we can voluntarily open those floodgates a bit at a time, and in a time of our choosing.

Make a commitment to honour what your body is experiencing in this instant and you will find that emotions begin to flow again. Once that flow begins, you may notice that energy spent repressing is now free, and that the energy that was repressed is also free. This leaves you free to use that energy as you choose, and to enjoy the ebb and flow of emotion, fearless and connected to this instant.

Day 3: Loving without Judgement

Great Expectations

The next barrier, expectation, gets in the way of human happiness every day. As soon as we get up in the morning, our expectations are ready to ruin our day if we get lost in them. If we wake up and expect there will be hot water for a shower and fuel in the car, if we expect that the car will get us to work, or the train will run on time, then we get angry and upset when any of those things don't happen – because life is not doing what we expect.

It may be worth defining expectations, which herein I describe differently to plans, goals or hopes. An expectation, as I define it, is a belief that something *should* happen, a belief that causes us pain when life and that 'should' don't quite line up. Goals and plans are fine, as long as they don't take on a stressful, compulsive quality; expectations, however, set us up for disappointment, anger and hurt.

Such expectations are bound to cause us trouble, because at some point, they will clash with reality – it's unavoidable. Unfortunately, reality does not adapt to our wishes. It has no interest in our expectations or in pleasing us. Reality runs its own race. It operates on cause and effect, and what happens is always what happens, without exception. Life is as it is. Flowers bloom, the sun shines, people are born and die, and at every step, humans fight with the happenings they disagree with. As we have seen already, it is these disagreements, and not the happenings themselves, that cause human suffering.

Think about people you know who are really unhappy, and notice how many unmet demands they make on life, including their jobs, their partners, the weather, etc. For example, people who are miserable at work generally have a lot of unmet expectations. They think they should be promoted, should earn more money, should be treated better, and so on. They think, they think, they think. They get lost in thinking they should have X, Y and Z, while life is giving them A, B and C and saying, 'Come on, this is what you need. Learn from this.'

Expectation closes us down because we have preconceived beliefs about how things should be; for instance, when I go to a restaurant, I should be greeted in this way, and the waiter should do such and such, and the food should come in this amount of time. Do you remember the expert's chair from Week 2? Well, experts always have expectations. Beginners just experience things. Now I'm not saying you should never complain. If things are not up to standard, you can tell people. But you can do that without forgetting about your happiness.

People who are stuck in their expectations can't enjoy life because they're too caught up in what it should and should not be. They can't experience life as it is. They are too fixated on thinking that life should change. I call this 'Should-ism', and it is the world's number one religion!

And when it comes to relationships, these 'shoulds' crank up several notches for a couple of important reasons. The first is that we believe that our loved ones are largely responsible for our happiness (or unhappiness). Examine your life, your behaviour or the behaviour of others, and this will become clear – we think that if others meet our expectations we will be happy and that if we aren't happy, it's because someone isn't doing their bit! The second reason for the expansion of 'shoulds' in close relationships is that the closer we are to someone, the better we know them, the more expertise we feel we have on their life and how they should live it.

Imagine you meet a stranger on the train and they tell you they just left their steady job to start a business, something they had always dreamed of doing. What would you say to them? Most of us would congratulate them and never think about that conversation again, because we have minimal expertise and no emotional investment. Now imagine your husband, wife or partner tells you they left their stable, predict-able job today and that they're going to start a new business, something they had always dreamed of. What would you say now? We would each respond differently to this depending on our financial situation, our tolerance of risk and how success-ful we believe the new business might be, but this becomes fertile ground for the 'shoulds' to run amok. Here are some possibilities:

- 'He should consult me before making big decisions like this.'
- 'She doesn't care about how this might affect me.'
- 'That was irresponsible. He should stick with his predictable job.'
- 'She shouldn't be so irresponsible.'

118 Mindfulness for Life

If these sorts of statements arise, we can be confident that an expectation has not been met, that judgement is getting in the way.

Activity: Dropping Judgement

Expectation is the same as judgement, which we talked about in detail in Week 2. The flip side of judgement, of course, is curiosity. The way to drop all expectation is to simply stay curious about the situation. This may be easier said than done, but it can be as simple as following your breath rather than getting caught up in your running thoughts. You can take a step out of the drama, your internal drama, and just breathe.

Try it right now. Feel your breath in your chest, and notice how it feels to breathe in and breathe out. Don't pay much attention to anything but the breath. As you do so, bring to mind a situation that has sparked stressful thinking and judgements about someone you love. Noticing the breath, watch those judgements arise and see if you can let them disappear without becoming involved in them. Simply let judgements fall back into the space they came from, and stay curious, breathing, wondering what comes next.

What if you could look upon your loved ones with this simple, grounded curiosity, free from judgement and expectation? You could still tell these people if you didn't like something they were doing, or you could still leave to find a more responsible, dependable partner. But you could leave in the spirit of: 'Darling, I love your adventurous spirit but it's not the life for me. I feel that a steady, dependable person is who I want to live with, and I don't want you to give up your dream. So I'm leaving. I love you and I hope it all works out.'

Or you might stay, enjoy the unpredictable ride and use it as a spark to bring to light your assumptions, expectations and judgements, an opportunity to know yourself better.

Either way, when it comes to relationships, there are only two choices: to live through expectation, which brings control and manipulation, or to live in the adventure of this instant, free to be and to let the other be, exactly as they are.

Day 4: Working without Thinking (Much)

Learning to Drop Thinking

Today, I will propose something fairly revolutionary; that you would be more successful at work if you didn't think so much. This may sound counter-intuitive because it is the opposite of popular wisdom. The standard line is that we need to be more thoughtful, more conscious and more planned when it comes to our actions at work, and there is some truth in that too.

Therefore it is important to separate practical, useful thinking (which I will call conscious thought) from the usual patterns of compulsive thinking. Conscious thought is the application of thought as a tool to solve problems and conceptualise new ideas. Thinking as we know it is an addiction to rumination, projection and reminiscing. It serves no purpose at work. On the contrary, compulsive thinking is detrimental to your work because, for every instant of rumination, you miss an opportunity to engage with this instant, and it is only in this instant that your best work can happen.

Conscious thought is a different beast, because it arises alongside conscious activity, rather than being a problem-solving strategy. When you are engaged in this instant, fresh thoughts can arise that are perfectly suited to the situation you find yourself in, while compulsive thinking can only regurgitate the past.

Consider this: imagine that you are deeply engaged in the solution of a complex problem, like solving a puzzle or inventing the light bulb. As you work, you focus on what you are doing, but thoughts keep coming up to distract you, thoughts like: 'You'll never figure it out. You might as well give up!' and 'What's for dinner?'

Whenever you lose yourself in these thoughts, you notice that energy drains away from the project, that your concentration is broken and that you feel stressed and anxious. On the other hand, when you simply focus on this step in the project, staying with the breath and connecting with the body, there is a calm, timeless quality about your work. And as you leave for the day to do something else, your subconscious mind keeps working on the problem, putting together possible solutions and eliminating them. Then, in a flash, an inspiring solution emerges from left field, something you would never have been able to figure out through the ordinary thinking process. By conscious thought, you allowed something new to enter the world through you.

Inspiration and Attention to Detail

Working in the present moment, inspiration could strike you at any time. And even when it doesn't, your work will be of a high quality because you will have attention to detail. When we are free of compulsive thinking, when we drop it altogether, we naturally become more attentive, we naturally pay closer attention to details that would not register when we are busy rushing to the imagined future. And it is in those tiny details that mastery happens and value is created.

Think of an open-heart surgeon, the best in the world. He or she has no more capability than you or I, but he is expert in performing delicate operations that require attention to minute details. You wouldn't like your surgeon trying to get through his work a little quicker in order to get an extra operation done, would you? And you wouldn't want him shaking and sweating because he was worried about killing you or failing the operation either. Instead, you want all his noticing and his nous fully engaged in your needs and your predicament in that instant.

And so the third barrier we need to drop is thinking itself, which may sound a little strange. How do you drop thinking? Well, we have already seen that there is a difference between compulsive thinking and conscious thought. Thought is something that arises of its own accord. It is a natural part of life. Thinking is the act of doing something with those thoughts, and of course, thinking can be very helpful at times. It can be quite useful and positive. At other times, however, it's an energy drain. It pulls you out of the present moment and causes you to dwell on the past and worry about the future. The act of thinking itself creates a barrier to being present in the moment.

Activity: Conscious Thought

How do you drop compulsive thinking and step into conscious thought? First, you need to be present, so take a moment now to use breath awareness or body awareness to bring your attention into the now. As you become present, direct your energy to a problem-solving activity, which could be a puzzle or it could be figuring out how to end a story you have been writing. Whatever the task, bring your total, conscious attention to the process, without concern for getting to the future in which the problem has been solved. Treat it like the creation of art, a process that is enjoyable in its own right, regardless of the result. Then, simply breathe, focus and engage: it's as simple as that. Be attentive to the thoughts that try to take your attention back into compulsive thinking.

By practising this process of not-thinking, you can get the best out of your mind without letting it cause you so many problems. I've found that my creativity, my job performance and all the things I do have improved as a result of learning not to think so much. I still get caught up in thought regularly – every day, in fact – but there are more and more times when I am just aware and watching, which has brought me enormous benefits. This approach allows creative insights to arise while ensuring conscientious, high-quality work on a consistent basis. Try it this week, and see how a small change in focus can make a big difference to your performance.

Let's consider that a little more. Thinking is the act of playing with thought. It is also the act of analysing life – trying to make sense of the things that happen, trying to fit them into categories and labelled boxes, and, finally, trying to use the analysis to eliminate past mistakes and create a perfect future. That is the mind's ultimate goal.

The Zen masters taught that to think not-thinking, think non-thinking; in other words, learn not to think. This is really a simple process. You move from swimming in thought, being lost in the fog, to watching it. This means bringing your attention into this moment, rather than daydreaming. If you take one mindful breath and feel your body from the inside, you will start to notice a sense of clarity and peace – this is what I mean by emerging from the fog. As thought takes over again, you may find yourself a million miles away, completely lost in that fog once more. Non-thinking means learning to watch thought come and go in a state of awareness, rather than losing yourself in that stream of thinking. As you continue to move between awareness and daydreams, you will notice the qualitative difference between these two states and your practice will continue to deepen.

Day 5: Living out of Control

Control is an Illusion

Today we will get a bit wild and creative, we will step outside of what's comfortable and we will engage in the world of unknowns from which all creativity emerges: the world of not knowing. The next barrier we need to drop is control. Our minds may scream and say, 'No, no, it's too dangerous.' But to move forward in life and in creativity, dropping control is a pre-requisite. Why? Because we don't have any. We have no control over the external world.

We tell ourselves stories to create the illusion of control, but in reality, we have none. For example, my mind tells me that I do my job really well, I am highly skilled, and ... story, story, story. That's how my mind assures me that I can keep my job and my income. But the reality is that next week the government of my country could decide the programme I work for is no longer needed, and I would be out of a job.

Or I could have a car accident and be unable to get up the stairs in my wheelchair, in which case I would no longer have a job, or I would have a different job. Likewise, I can work really hard, but whether I get a pay raise is not in my control. Regardless of how I try to line my ducks up and get them in an orderly row, I don't have control over things.

In fact, we need to drop the illusion that we have control in the first place and we need to let go of any attempt to wrest control from the world.

Dancing with Life

We might picture ourselves, and every creature in this world, as dancing with life (and life is definitely in the lead). We can respond to that lead in different ways, but we are not in control of the dance itself. Life can be joyful and graceful if we go with life, and it can be clunky, jerky and downright painful if we try to fight against it.

For example, a friend told me a story recently about a friend who lost her job. She was distraught at the time and worried about her income, quality of life and career direction. A year later, successful in a new venture, she reported back to my friend that it was 'the best decision I never made'. This person moved beyond the fear of losing the old, embraced the dance and was successful in the new direction in which life pushed her.

I am sure that you also have experienced changes you did not want at the time, but that led to positive growth and new opportunities that you would not have considered had you not been forced. Consider the boyfriend or girlfriend you wanted to marry in high school and who you are thankful you don't live with now. Remember the job you missed out on right before your dream job came along. And, every day, notice the opportunities that arise when the mind's desires are thwarted.

Becoming a Better Dance Partner

Before life drags us in a new direction, it usually gives a few subtle nudges and some gentle guidance. If we become attuned to these early directions, it is possible to flow with life's direction without needing such large shocks (although they may still happen at times). You can actively listen for life's wisdom and in the process you can unlock your hidden creativity. Here's how:

Activity: Listening for Direction

Is there a decision that feels right to you, but that you have been avoiding? Is there something you wish you could do more of, or do differently, if only you weren't afraid? Or is life giving you a nudge that you are steadfastly ignoring in the hope that you can cling to the old and familiar?

> Take a pen and paper and spend a few minutes follow-
> ing your breath while you write the answer to this question:
> if life could give me some advice, what would it be?
> Take as long as you need to complete your list, and if
> nothing comes, simply sit, breathe and be open to what-
> ever guidance could arise, whether it does or not.

Control or Influence?

This talk of dancing with life, listening for direction may
well raise the question: 'Don't we have any control?' Well, of
course, our behaviour and our choices affect things, so perhaps we could say we have some influence. But even if we do
everything 'right', we ultimately don't have control, even on a
small scale. And if the climate warms too much and sea levels
rise and all these other things happen, our lives will be out of
control in ways far beyond our jobs, relationships, etc.

The idea of being out of control brings up a lot of fear
because you have always believed that you have some control,
and you think that's what is keeping you safe right now. You
think that's what keeps things running smoothly. But the
truth is that our attempts to control are actually blocking us.
Trying to control gets in the way of fully connecting with life
as it is, which is where the real magic starts to happen.

When you drop the perception that you have control over
outcomes, and focus on where you have influence – which is
in responding to the moment as best you can – you can truly
start to dance with life. You start to get in the flow. When
that happens, things do tend to go well (though not always).

But when we drop the illusion of control, things start to flow much better.

Today I invite you to enjoy that flow, and to let the wisdom of the universe do the rest.

Day 6: Dropping the Burden of Good Health

Embracing Your True Health

Good health, a burden? What a crazy concept! It would seem that good health is a necessity for a happy life, that it is a prerequisite to contentment of any kind. But, in fact, it is a great burden, something that causes stress, anxiety, fear and distraction, and something you should drop as quickly as you can. Let me explain.

My friend Joan (not her real name) is always breaking down physically. She has an ache here, a cold there, some tendonitis and that slipped disc from back in the sixties. I know this because she tells me so, regularly and loudly, almost whenever I see her. But Joan suffers not because of the ailments she describes, but because of the belief that leads her to talk about them so frequently, the belief that is hidden under all those complaints: the belief that she should be healthy. Joan, like many of us, has fallen victim to the belief that her body should work better, that her health should improve, and that life was meant to be pain-free.

As we have seen throughout this journey so far, it is not the ailments that cause us to suffer, but the belief that it should be different, and health is an area of life in which this rings especially true. In the modern West, there is increasingly a perception that life should go on, largely pain-free, for as long as I'd like. Death is still fairly taboo, and the images we see in the media make it clear to the thinking mind (which absorbs this without question) that ageing has no place in our lives, that we should remain eternally young. The message is clear: you should be young, healthy and fit, otherwise there is something wrong.

As you may have noticed, the belief that there is something wrong is a very stressful thing, as it feeds those two painful processes – the struggle with what is and the search for happiness in the future – that cause our suffering. And as you may also have noticed, your body is exactly as it is right this instant, no matter how much you complain about it.

Activity: True Health

The only true health is being healthy in body and mind right now. What else is there but a story, a thought about the future? While Joan expends mental and physical energy arguing with her circumstances, I invite you to spend a few minutes in the only true health: one healthy instant. Now, one healthy instant does not require any particular physical or mental condition, it doesn't indicate that you need to be free of stress or aches or pains, just that you find a healthy connection to now. Try it with me …

Take a breath, whether short or long, easy or wheezy, and feel this instant moving, lungs, air, chest, just feel that. Smile as you breathe and notice your physical and mental state with a caring ease – not distant, but not worried about any imbalances – breathe, smile and let this body be.

For a few minutes, let any thoughts about future health float by undisturbed, and do the same for any thoughts of future illness. They're just thoughts after all, and with or without them this body is as it is right this second, so breathe, smile and enjoy. Close your eyes and smile at your body from the inside, act as if it is doing the best it can (which it is) and show your appreciation with a smile and a conscious breath. Spend a few minutes thanking your body for life's adventure (so far) through this simple, joyful process.

Today is your opportunity to find a realistic path to good health, which is only possible right now. That path, like all true ones, is the opposite of what you have been taught, which is to think about, worry about and plan for the health of this body. But let me be clear; I am not suggesting you stop taking care of this body, or that you stop scheduled medical checks. Take the best care you can of this body, not only through life-style choices but by freeing it of the incredible strain of future projection. Make the best choices you can in this instant and if a health challenge arises, embrace it. This sounds crazy per-haps, but what choice do you have? This health challenge is a part of your experience of this life, something the universe intended you to have, otherwise how could it be? And even if you think it is unfair, unjust or that you should have prevented it, it's here! Why not treat this challenge as another part of the adventure called life? Will you survive? Who knows? But your happiness cannot survive a fight with this instant, and besides being happy and at peace, what purpose have we in this body?

These challenges can become a gift on your journey of waking up if you take note of the mind's resistance, if you watch the fight with what is, and if you learn to sit, breathe and smile.

You can experience the best health possible right now by letting the concept of perfect health drift past. It sounds paradoxical, but it's true: the more you want some ideal that doesn't exist now, the more you suffer, while total acceptance of this body, doing its best in this instant, is enough to bring peace, and what could be more healthy than that.

Day 7: Living Mindfully: Life as a happening

Letting Your Life Flow

Dropping all barriers will bring you back to curiosity, freedom, interest and not-thinking. Your identity will fade into the background, and your life will flow with ease. There is no way to describe this experience adequately, so I hope you will experience it yourself instead.

You do not need to become anything else, learn anything new or gain extra wisdom to live in this way. It is simply a matter of dropping the barriers standing in the way of your true nature. Begin by dropping expectations, and picking up curiosity instead.

Often our expectations about the world are hidden, even from ourselves. But life does a brilliant job of uncovering these expectations by giving us plenty of situations that aren't what we want, thus providing us with great practice. When the food comes out cold, and you feel anger and frustration rising, you don't have to change the way you deal with the situation – but be curious.

Spend some time breathing and noticing your physical reaction. Notice the thoughts that go along with it and the way the thoughts and physical sensations feed each other. Bringing curiosity to the situation allows you to become aware of those debilitating expectations. Situations that seem wrong can become learning opportunities or chances to try something different. Potentially, they can even become positive experiences.

Without fixed expectations, you will be able to find opportunities where there seem to be none. You will become a master problem-solver because you can stay curious and engaged when others become frustrated, and you will become the wonderful friend, family member and partner you are capable of being, as you allow the other to be as they are. In this, you drop expectations, as well as identity because you are dropping the big one: thinking.

Activity: Dropping Thinking by Watching Thoughts

You can do that now. Take your attention to the breath, and watch what thoughts the mind is producing right now. Watch them as they come and go. Enjoy the process. Treat the thoughts as if they were people walking past your house. You can see them, you can hear them and you can watch them coming and going, but there is no need to chase them. There is no need to play with them, try to change them or get rid of them. You can just notice them.

Those thoughts aren't you, nor are they yours, they just are. Instead of following the habitual path of becoming entranced by thought, you can retain your place as the watcher, the one who sees thoughts come and go.

A big part of learning not to think is making the shift from paying attention to the content of thoughts, which is what we do normally, to paying attention to the process of watching the thoughts. We step from being fascinated by what the thoughts are saying to being interested in the process of watching them come and go. We're not caught up in what they say and what they mean and whether it's true or not. We step out of all of that and enjoy the show instead!

Spend a few minutes enjoying the show now. Use breath awareness to stay anchored in the now, and as you do so let those thoughts arise and disappear in their own time.

Life as a Happening

As you watch thought, you come to the realisation there is no Me here. There's no firm identity. There's no one keeping you alive when you're not thinking about it. It's just happening. The body keeps breathing; the mind keeps thinking; the feet keep moving; the heart keeps beating. Obviously, the brain is sending out impulses that tell the organs and the muscles what to do. But there is no 'you' steering the ship and making it all happen. You are there, and you get to watch it and enjoy it or get lost in the bits and pieces. You get to have the adventure. Some of the adventure is in the land of story, and some of it is in the land of awareness.

Most people treat life like a race, or a competition – you against life – but what happens still happens. And what is life but this instant, a cool breeze, a squawking bird, the honk of a car horn? Everything else is just my story. The only reality is in this instant, is this instant. So I ask you, my dear friend: do you want to race and compete until this body dies? Or will you embrace the happening that is life, the only life, right this second? The choice may be small, but the difference is immense.

WEEK 6

Waking Up Now!

This week is all about waking up, but not in the conventional sense. When we wake up every morning, our state of consciousness changes, and with it our experience. We move from a dream world to a world of people, places, things and reality. And when we move into this world, the world of the dream no longer makes sense and no longer seems important – even though 15 minutes earlier, that dream may have caused fear, anger, joy or despair. Regardless of the dream's power while we were asleep, and no matter how vivid it may have been, we know in the awakened state that it doesn't matter a bit.

But what most people don't realise is that human beings don't leave dreams behind when we get out of bed – we just stop recognising them as dreams. After all, what is a thought but a story or an image arising in the mind? What is the world created through thinking but a fantasy told by you, perhaps 'based on a true story'? If you feel that this is confrontational, or that it seems to be an odd way to describe what we normally see as 'fact', I completely understand.

I went through years of believing my thoughts, years of

being convinced that my viewpoint was right and was true. But what I realised when I woke up out of that dream was that the thoughts and stories flowing through my mind moment after moment were no more than imaginings. I recognised that although certain things do happen, the meaning I make from those events is a story all of my own. But, most importantly, I noticed that being lost in these stories kept me focused on the outside world – focused on the events around me and dependent on them for my happiness. What I want for you is what I have access to now: the ability to wake up out of these dreams and into the real world, which is always kinder than what the mind describes. This world is a wonderful place.

This week, we will explore the process of waking up and I will share some simple ways to speed this process up. As the term 'waking up' implies, we are not making this process happen, we are simply setting the conditions to support it.

Awake but Dreaming

Imagine yourself in a beautiful place on a beautiful day. Maybe it's that beach in Thailand or the south of France. Wherever you are, picture that place in your mind and add one more detail: tomorrow you will find out whether you will lose your job in a company restructure. Where would your attention be focused? On the beautiful surroundings? Or on the imagined future? Every time your attention wandered to those thoughts about unemployment, poverty and despair, you would enter the dream world I am describing, imagining a problematic future and losing the one thing you can enjoy: the present moment. Of course, you could also wake up at any moment and re-engage with the world around you right now.

For most mindfulness students, life is a journey that moves between the dream world (thinking) and the real world (your experience now), and our practice is a way to strengthen this present-moment awareness, while loosening the grip of that thought-based dream world.

Nothing to Attain

If you set aside time to formally practise every day, that practice will contribute a little more energy to waking up. That is all we are doing. If your mind needs to have some goal in order just to sit, that's fine, but don't measure your practice by any goal – including the goal to develop certain qualities, improve your self-esteem or become something.

Don't measure your practice by anything – just sit and experience it. Sit and breathe and look and listen and feel yourself doing that. Notice who is doing that. That is all there is to the practice.

The usefulness of anything you do or learn or read can be measured by whether it helps you wake up or helps you stay asleep. And sometimes, experiences that we like can help us stay asleep. As you notice the experiences or relationships that deepen your slumber, you may find yourself doing something different.

When I first started practising meditation, I sometimes used it as a way to stay asleep and to strengthen my thought-based identity. I could say, 'Now I'm a meditation student,' or 'I'm a Buddhist,' or 'I'm a Zen practitioner. I know all this stuff and I've read all these books that you haven't read so I'm pretty amazing.'

And it was all made up. It was all stories in my head. It was another attempt to find happiness and peace outside – this time through Buddhism or books or becoming this or turning into that.

Now I read books that wake me up, that resonate and that help me reach a state of awareness more easily. I will rarely read a whole book at once. I may read a few pages and then, once I am awake, I go about my day, or I go to sleep at night (meaning physical sleep, not lost-in-thought sleep). I use what's around me. I use experiences to remind me to wake up, rather than using them to stay asleep or to hide from myself.

Normally, most of us look outside ourselves for happiness. We are always in search of the ideal situation – the perfect place to live, the perfect job, more money or better relationships. We want people to think well of us, and we want people to be nice to us. We have all these expectations and desires, and we think that if those are fulfilled, we'll find happiness. We live in the hope that someday the outside world is going to fulfil us.

Missing Out on Life

We don't experience the moment or the inner world because thinking is going on all the time, and we are so caught up in it that we can't experience our lives – we can't sense ourselves there in the background. Thought is so powerful, so hypnotising to humans, that we can't sense our own aliveness. How crazy is that? It's insanity.

It is as though you lived your life to the age of 40 or 50 before you realised you had hands. All that time, you thought they were missing because you never looked. Then finally, you looked down and realised, 'Hmm, I've got hands. Wow, isn't that amazing? I had hands the whole time. I never looked!' Of course, you would laugh!

The Agony and the Irony

We are all running around looking outside for this thing that has been in us the whole time. And everything that has happened in our lives is pushing us to wake up – every frustration, every disappointment, every joy. Life is saying to us every day, every second, 'Wake up, wake up, wake up! Look inside, look inside, look inside!'

And mostly, we say, 'No, I don't want to. I want to look over there. There's something shiny there. That grass is greener. I don't want to look inside because it's scary, and I don't know what I might find. I am going to take another look over there first.'

That's OK; it doesn't matter. It doesn't matter at all. It doesn't matter whether anyone wakes up to this or not, because it is who we are. It is the energy that drives the universe, and it's not going anywhere. It doesn't have any timeline we need to follow. Our evolution occurs as we slowly wake up out of this thought, and out of this thought, and out of thinking itself.

Day 1: Waking Up to Yourself

Finding Space, Ending Drama

Certain things will happen this week if you practise the exercises every single day. First, you will notice some space between you and thought, which leads to a more sceptical view of those mental stories. I sometimes call this 'waking up to yourself', because that noticing of the space between you and thought is the first step in illuminating who you really are. The power of thought comes from its ability to grab your attention – like a good movie or TV show – and from your wholehearted engagement in the dream world. Even beyond that, thought gets its power from the fact that you identify with it, you believe the thought is you.

When we completely believe stories to be true, the pictures they paint (which are often of a scary future or an unfair past) provoke emotions that increase our engagement in the story. And once we are hooked, it is as hard to step back from those thoughts as it is to turn off a thriller ten minutes before the end. But before you're hooked, it's quite easy to switch it off. It's quite easy to walk past without engaging in the drama.

As you wake up this week, you will start to get off the hook, you will start to notice that some of the 'facts' of your life are actually opinions. You will notice that some things you hold to be true are no more than beliefs, and that some of your problems have no reality right now, but are merely things that might happen in the future. You have probably started to experience this already.

Moving to the Inner World

The second thing you will notice, as you wake up out of thought, is that your attention will naturally move more and more from the outside world to the inside world. That doesn't mean you will disconnect from what's outside, but you will stop looking there for what's important. In essence, you take care of your inner state first. And when you seem to have a problem, you focus on that inner world first, paying attention to what is arising inside right now.

Doing this puts the power in your hands because you realise that the outside world has no control over your happiness. As you return inside and wake up again and again, it becomes clear that being lost in thought is the only barrier to joy right now.

Activity: Waking Up to Awareness

Go inside now, and feel the breath coming and going. Try to drop your attention into the chest. Notice all the things going on there – movement, feelings, thoughts coming and going – but also notice who is watching. Who is there watching all those things happening and noticing as they arise and disappear?

There is no answer to that question. Rather than trying to answer it, I invite you to sit with the question. Who is there inside? Who is watching? Of course, the mind may come up with all kinds of answers that make logical sense, but as we've discovered already, they don't make experiential sense. When you actually look for the elements of identity, you can't catch them. You can't find them. But we know that we exist, and that's enough.

So stay with that. Notice a strange phenomenon: you can stay inside while still opening your eyes and taking in what's outside. It is a curious thing that you can actually see the outside world more clearly when your attention is focused inside.

> Take your attention deeper and deeper into that inner world and allow it to harmonise with the outside world. The harmonising happens naturally; you don't have to do anything. Feel the body from the inside, sense yourself as awareness, and then look around. You can get up and walk and talk; you can breathe and go to work and do other things. But there's a vortex of peace that surrounds you when you come from that inner space.

When I realised that my true identity is the awareness underneath all my conditioning, thoughts and physical form, it was like waking up from a stressful dream. It means that if this body has problems or needs treatment, the problem isn't 'mine' (although I make sure it's taken care of as well as possible), it is simply a situation that needs my attention. And as all the other problems I used to see as 'mine', be they financial, social or otherwise, lost that sense of ownership (because after this body dies they will be no more), my life has become unimaginably simple. Paradoxically, since this shift began, I am managing money, health and relationships far better than I ever did when they were 'my problem'.

No Belongings

This voice doesn't belong to me, this body doesn't belong to me, and none of that matters. The interesting thing is that as I continue to wake up, I realise that it doesn't even matter whether I wake up or not. And I realise that the stress I experience by being asleep isn't actually enduring or real – it is invented through thought.

Of course, stress feels real at the time. But when you know yourself as this background of awareness, you also know that when the body dies, it's not the end of that awareness. Once you sense that it doesn't matter whether your body dies, your stress doesn't matter either.

Finding True Peace

As we close, shift your attention to the breath once more, and notice who it is that is breathing. Thought may still be there, but notice that when you step out of thinking and just breathe and look around, it feels peaceful.

The body may not be peaceful. There may be a lot of emotion and sensation flying around, but peace is there in the background. It is who you are. Experience that, and continue to come back to it. My whole teaching is to stop thinking and to experience instead – particularly to experience yourself. That is the whole practice.

Now it is up to you. Are you ready to wake up? Has it already started? I think it has. Do you want to use your everyday experiences, your stress, or whatever arises to wake you up out of this dream, this nightmare, of thought? Or do you need to sleep a little longer? That's OK too. We are not really asleep; we have just forgotten.

Once you start to wake up, you will realise there is nothing to accomplish, there is no rush and there is no time either. You can enjoy this process that is happening through you. And, in that, there is true peace, relaxation and total contentment. It doesn't get any better.

Day 2: The Gift of Challenge

Mindfulness and Alarm Clocks

The world will give you all these experiences to remind you to wake up. It will give you experiences that cause frustration and stress. You will feel anger arising, and you will get lost in thought. Everything that's part of human history will play out inside you. Getting lost in thinking or drama or combat is our history. It's our collective conditioning, and it's all moving through you. How cool is that?

There's nothing you need to do but look at yourself and sense yourself as the watcher. Keep feeling yourself in the background watching. That's hard to do when you're lost in thought. So come back to the breath, and ask yourself who is noticing the breath. Don't answer – just sit with the question. Who is watching?

I experience the peace of waking up quite regularly, even though I don't always feel peaceful. And there is nothing special about me – far from it. I am as ordinary as can be. But I do know that place inside, and I do come from that place to some extent, and my experience of that place gets stronger every day. I sometimes call it remembering, but it feels more like waking up.

With each experience, each thing I read, and each practice, I feel as though the alarm clock is going off again. I'm being reminded that I am not those thoughts and I'm not this experience – that the identity I take on and the role I play during the day isn't who I am.

Stress and the Outside World

I use stress as a reminder that I have fallen asleep once more and that the alarm clock is going off again. This helps me to realise that I don't need to seek experiences that make me happy. Of course, we don't need to seek experiences that make us unhappy, but there will always be something that rubs us up the wrong way because we put so many demands on life.

It is inevitable that the outside world will frustrate and disappoint our minds. The world is full of seven billion people all chasing what they want – all believing that if they get certain things, if they have certain experiences and if their lives look a certain way, they will be happy. Of course there is going to be conflict out there. If we are living in that whirlpool, we are going to get swirled around a bit.

But when we can step out of that and into waking up, the situations that conflict with what we want become tools for practice. They become incredibly simple, powerful ways to continue to wake up. We can realise that our experience in that whirlpool, or what we call 'my life', is really a bunch of thoughts about many separate experiences. Every morning I go to work, and in my mind and my memory, it seems very similar every day. But if I am paying attention, every day is completely different. My body is different, the air is different and everything around me is different from what it was even the day before.

But the mind doesn't notice that. It connects things and creates patterns. Each day I go to work and have a completely different experience, but my mind creates a story that says, 'My work is like this, and my colleague is like this.' Then the mind looks for evidence to support that story. Ample research has shown that once you have come to a conclusion about something, your mind will look for and focus on the evidence that supports your existing story, and will ignore the things that don't support it.

Today, you can embrace a new way to deal with stress, seeing it not as an enemy but as a pushy friend, who won't let you get away with snoozing on. What would happen, how would your life experience change, if you used every little upset, every frustration, to come back to the present moment? Emotions are often seen as something needing to be pushed aside or clung to, depending on whether they are 'good' or 'bad', but as we have seen, this leads only to a life of confusion and struggle. If we are to lead a life of peace, it is necessary to wake up to this pattern and engage in a different way with these pushy friends.

When that ball appears in your stomach, or your face feels all flushed from embarrassment, use it as a reminder. Ask yourself the question: what am I avoiding? What am I unwilling to embrace? Then let your attention explore whatever is inside.

As soon as you begin this process, the grip of thought loosens, life becomes less of a struggle and the path of peace becomes clear: just the step in front of you, just now.

Day 3: Relationships are a Mindfulness Practice

Waking Up from 'Shoulds'

Every human who is yet to fully wake up lives with the same delusion: you should be different! That 'you' could be your mother, your brother, your boss, anyone you see as an 'other'. And the ways in which they should be different can be many and varied, from being kinder, to more confident, to more obedient, to more anything. The qualities and the people involved are interchangeable, but the underlying structure is the same. In essence, it is the fight with this instant, framed from a different perspective. Those people are a part of the present moment, so the suggestion that they should be different indicates that this instant should be different too!

Let me repeat (because it's important) that because of the structure of this pattern, the people and the 'shoulds' are interchangeable. If those people did change, the mind would look for a new dissatisfaction, because it is dissatisfaction that it seeks! Your mind is not looking for contentment, it is looking for a problem to fix! Whatever happens, the misery is there. Even if you could train everyone to do exactly what you wanted, when you wanted, always, the misery would remain.

This is an innocent misunderstanding. The mind believes that problem-solving is the path to happiness, when in fact it is the only obstacle to experiencing that happiness right this instant! The unhappiness that the structure produces shows us that this structure is unhelpful, and ironically that's a very helpful thing to realise! And so, relationships (which when experienced through the mind are a source of pain) become a rich field for mindfulness practice.

It turns out that a partner who is difficult may be the best kind and a boss who gives you grief could be the finest of all! There is a radical shift in perspective taking place here and it is worth spelling out. The old way was to assume that the world's responsibility is to make me happy. The world, from this viewpoint, should provide what I want, give me pleasant experiences and generally do as I tell it. As the world is responsible for my happiness, it is also to blame for my unhappiness, as it is not giving me the things that it should. This way of living leaves me as the powerless victim (or beneficiary) of life's fortunes, and in that role, arguing with life may be the only thing that gives me some sense of power! Much of this complaining revolves around relationships with other humans (who are stuck in the same pattern) and so it seems that other people are obstacles to peace.

The new way of being and seeing requires me to take full responsibility for my own state of happiness or unhappiness. Because I know that happiness arises from a deep connection with myself and this moment, my relationship to challenges can be completely different. From this point of view, every frustration, disappointment and so-called disaster is an opportunity to wake up once more. Knowing that you could never give me happiness or disturb my peace (only my thinking can do that), you are free to be who you are and I don't need you to change a thing. You become my teacher, showing me where I am stuck and helping trigger the signal (stress) that lets me know I have fallen asleep once more.

The distance between these two states is incredibly narrow, but the *difference* between them is enormous. This shift can move us from relationships of dependence and drama to free, loving connections because it takes all the fear and neediness out of our interactions. When you wake up to the fact that others aren't supposed to make you happy, freedom is yours to enjoy.

Activity: Mindful Mentors

Ironically, the least mindful people in your life may be your greatest teachers, because they will draw out the reactions driven by stuck old mind patterns, they will bring to the surface past emotional pain, and they can (if you watch them) illustrate the insanity of the human mind! We should thank these people.

To skilfully use these mindfulness aids, we must be deliberate and conscious. Take a moment now to think of someone who raises a strong reaction in you: a relative, friend, co-worker, politician, it doesn't really matter. It would be best to pick someone you have regular contact with, so you can notice the strong reactions that may arise in their presence.

Notice what happens in your body and mind when you think of them. Don't get involved in the *content* of the story, just watch the pattern emerging. Breathe, smile and stay conscious as you watch this pattern.

Spend a few minutes sitting with those emotions and thoughts. Make friends with them. And next time you see that person, see if you can stay present, watchful and breath-focused. If reactions still arise, there's more work to do, and those mindfulness aids will show you where that work is.

Day 4: Awakened Work

Hiding in Work

My friend Jodie almost breathes work, you can smell it on her, even at weekends. She works with an anxious quality, checks emails when she is sick or on holiday and acts as if the whole company would implode if she didn't check that one last email on Sunday night. But it's not the Protestant work ethic or a deep sense of duty that drives Jodie to these lengths. The truth of the matter is that Jodie is hiding. She is hiding from the questions that arise when she can't define herself by her work, questions like 'Who am I really?' She is hiding from the unease that she experiences in a moment that isn't filled with tasks and stimuli. And most of all, Jodie is hiding from herself. She is scared to find out what is there underneath thought and activity. (What if there's nothing?)

Jodie uses work to stay asleep, frightened as she is of waking up from the dream, and maybe you do too. Many people find an identity in a job, a role in life, and that identity, though unsatisfying, gives them *something* to think about, talk about and be. Of course this creates stress and dissatisfaction eventually, so the waking-up process still works; everything other than waking up eventually leads to pain. But used consciously, your job can be both a contribution to this world and a help on your mindfulness journey.

Mindful Work Practice

Let's say for a moment that your only true job for this lifetime was to wake up out of thinking. Imagine that there was nothing else you want to achieve in this lifetime (although you might like to try a few experiences along the way), and that your place of work provided a place to wake up (as the workplace will bring up the stressful thinking that keeps you asleep). How would this change your relationship to your work? Imagine if being present while working became more important than the type of work you do, who you work for or how much you are paid. Imagine if the quality you brought into each task by working mindfully, peacefully, was more important than the end result of that work. This shift is an amazing experience.

A few years ago I made a conscious shift. I noticed that work was becoming a means to an end, or something I wanted to escape by starting my own business, being able to work from home and having as much time as I wanted with my kids. And each time I hatched an escape plan, I felt happy and excited for a while, until it failed to materialise. And then I wondered: what if I am in this job in this place at this time because I am supposed to be in this job in this place at this time? What if it is an opportunity rather than a barrier? And so I decided to make mindfulness my only aim at work. I started paying closer attention to how I did my work, instead of arguing with life. I gave my fullest attention to engaging in the process of what I do, without worrying about the end result. And I used every stress as a reminder, every challenge as an opportunity to become more present.

The change has been a remarkable one, bringing many unexpected benefits. I became better at my job, more success-ful in my career and in each role, and my enjoyment of the work steadily increased. But all these, I later realised, were mere side effects. The true benefit is twofold: work makes me more mindful and through work I bring mindfulness into the world. Every day at work becomes a meditation retreat, an opportunity to realise who I am. And every minute in which I bring peace into the world, it spreads. I often drift into thinking during the day but those glimpses seem to be enough to create a spark in those around me.

But underneath all these benefits is my true selfish motive: I want to be at peace. If you make this your main driver, it changes everything.

Activity: Peace at Work

Close your eyes for a few minutes and imagine a day at work with a difference. Imagine that your only true concern is your internal state, and that your only aim during the day is to be present. Take a mindful breath to remember what that is like, then continue to imagine. Picture yourself working your way through the day with this single focus. How would you walk, talk and sit? How important would the usual daily dramas become? And what might your experience be like? Take some time to explore.

Reflect for a moment on a simple truth: every task you complete, everything you do and everything you create has a lifespan. Eventually it will be gone. What will remain in the next job, the next experience? Just you. Your to-do list from ten years ago is dead, as is last week's. The only lasting, fulfilling achievement for any human is unconditional peace. Rather than a life of busy work and striving towards an empty task list, use it to find contentment, peace and joy.

Today, I invite you to test this approach and see what happens. You may find yourself in a world of ease and contentment, even in that place we're not supposed to enjoy – the place we call 'work'.

Day 5: Life is an Adventure

The End of Problems

As you wake up into this instant, you will experience an acuteness, a joyfulness and a sense of curiosity in your everyday life. You will find that life becomes an adventure to be enjoyed instead of a problem to be solved. Adventure always happens now, while problems always exist in the past or the future. And as you wake up from thought, you are waking up out of the past and the future into the present moment. Naturally, the experience of being here now is infinitely more enjoyable than a life lost in thought.

Discovering that life is an adventure, not a puzzle or a maths problem, is the beginning of the awakening of your creative self, a side of you that may have been battered, ignored and denied for years while the thinking mind was busy chewing over the same problems, seeking a logical solution. Today I invite you to let that side loose a little, and to see the adventure that every day can be.

Becoming an Adventurer

It is possible to experience life as an adventure if you step, for an hour or two, into the shoes of an adventurer, a role that has some very different characteristics to normal, everyday human existence. First of all, an adventure is a mystery. You don't know what you will find, so good adventurers are careful to keep their expectations in check, lest they block some new discovery. Adventurers seek out and embrace this mystery, looking for possibilities where others see none. They keep a lively curiosity about them when exploring so that new openings can be recognised and investigated, and lastly they bring a sense of wonder to all that is around them.

The creative person applies the same approach to life, even in seemingly familiar places and situations. They bring a deep curiosity about the way the world works, an interest in the world around them and they pay close attention to that world, allowing new ideas and possibilities to show themselves. You can be an adventurer too.

Activity: Today's Adventure

Today is no ordinary day; it is a day like no other. It will never be repeated, remixed or replayed on catch-up. When this day ends, it will be the close of 24 hours never to be seen again, so please don't drift through it. Instead, today I ask you to make it your mission to explore the world around you as if you had never been there before. Here are some simple ways to step into this space:

1. Sit, breathe mindfully and visually explore your surroundings. Look around as if you had never seen any of the objects around you before. Study them in detail, notice as much as you can about them and keep breathing, lest you lose that curiosity in thought.

2. Sit and listen to your surroundings for a few minutes. Close your eyes and listen intently, treating each sound as if you had never heard it before. You may want to breathe mindfully to keep focused on this instant.

3. When walking a familiar path today (this could be the route to work or simply through your hall) combine the two activities listed above and see what you notice. Listen and look as if you just landed on this planet with the mission of noticing as much as you can while you're here.

Once you have had a taste of this curious space, apply it to ordinary, everyday situations, like doing the dishes or completing tasks at work. Apply your attention well, and see what new things you notice and what arises through this process.

Creative breakthroughs often happen not because of some vast genius or intelligence, but because we learn to pay careful attention to the world around us. And whether this creativity comes in the form of art, invention or seeing through an old pattern of behaviour that no longer serves you, the noticing is the most important element. In any situation or human interaction, the old way sustains itself because no one (or not enough people) spots the pattern and sees through it to a new way. Most of us either don't notice, or get stuck on complaining about the old way, reinforcing its power through resistance. If instead you can become intimate with those situations and patterns, like the response you keep getting from your mother when you tell her to take better care of herself, or the way your workplace wastes energy and time through pointless meetings, a new option may well emerge. And when you bring forth this new option with a curious, adventurous attitude, others are much more likely to embrace what you bring.

Imagine yourself bringing a new idea to a colleague, friend or family member with this sort of attitude. Picture yourself explaining this idea with that spirit of wonder and curiosity, open to their perspective and with no agenda in mind. How would that feel? And what sort of response might you get? Allow this natural curiosity to awaken and every conversation becomes an opportunity to notice something new.

Hone this noticing and you will become energised, engaged and enthusiastic about this incredible world, and who knows what happens next?

Day 6: Natural Wellness

True Gratitude

The only wellness is a present moment well lived. All else is a thought in your head. You have no future, and no past. You were born this instant in this place, so why complicate things with so much thinking? You are intensely healthy already, but you miss it because you are too busy worrying, thinking, planning and scheming to notice. So today, I ask you, please stop it! Drop all this ridiculous imagining of something non-existent, and instead notice the deep, abiding wellness that you have at your fingertips right now.

This may sound easy, and it is, although the mind has momentum and will likely return. That's OK. Take a step back from thinking for a second and you will notice some interesting facts. First, the body is keeping you alive, by breathing, pumping blood and regulating thousands of other systems, even when you are daydreaming, even when you are asleep! Second, the world around you is providing you with exactly what you need to stay alive for another moment. The earth maintains its orbit, the sun continues exploding, the winds move, the oceans pulse and the mix of oxygen stays at the ideal level for your uniquely formed lungs and heart. Finally, you did nothing to deserve any of this, you didn't create it and you can't make it continue, you are completely helpless. If the sun runs out of energy, or the earth falls out of orbit, nothing will survive. The universe creates these ideal circumstances for you, moment after moment, and what do humans do? Complain about the cold, moan that we should be richer, grizzle about the food being slow at the restaurant. We're an ungrateful lot.

Activity: Grateful Wellness

Close your eyes and take a long slow breath, smiling at the same time. As you breathe out, enjoy the sensation, let your shoulders drop and relax. Soak up the wonder of life, experiencing the feeling of breathing one more time as this life continues. Use that smile to thank the world for the oxygen, the body for the energy and the universe for the remarkable series of coincidences that allowed you to ever exist in the first place.

As the breath continues, feel the energy of the body from the inside and notice the way the energy pulsates through the hands, the feet and the body as a whole. Sit, breathe, feel the body and smile as you notice the deep wellness that is there in this instant, regardless of the body's state of wellbeing. Let the physical body relax into this thankfulness, but don't worry about any residual stress in the muscles or the joints, just sink into this instant and enjoy it. Take as long as you like to enjoy this state. Stay there for the rest of your life if you like!

As you wake up to the wellness that goes beyond physical or mental health, gratitude is natural. Underneath all the superficial happenings of your life, physical health, material wealth or poverty and all the other circumstances with which human beings concern themselves, there is a deep peace, an incredible wellness. In moments of flow, in which we embrace life wholeheartedly, seemingly because of some outside experience, like an amazing concert or breathtaking natural beauty, this deep connection sometimes shows itself. If you remember the standout moments of your life – the birth of your children, the day you got married, the trip to Spain – you were in this flow. The moment seemed so complete, so powerful or so important that everyday problems disappeared and you were able to notice what is always there – you!

Afterwards, you probably thought the experience was the key to what you felt. You thought that it was childbirth, or Spain, or the Rolling Stones that brought you into this state, which is true in some ways. The experience created an opening in your thought stream, a gap in which ordinary thinking was seen to be as unimportant as it is. And when those issues your mind chews over every day were illuminated as being completely irrelevant, something else was able to emerge. The life force that is you, that which only just battles to the surface through the layers of mental fog, was given the space to emerge and show itself. The external happenings helped, as a crack in a dam wall allows the great waters above to burst free, but isn't the creator of those waters.

So too, anything that seems to create deep peace and contentment is merely helping to remove some barriers, to make a space for that peace, or to draw that state out. This book might serve this purpose for some, as it resonates with that state of happiness that is as natural as the air we breathe, but that remains hidden under the conditioning of the human mind. Likewise, stress and disaster can cause old beliefs to crumble, leaving an uncertain space in which our natural, mindful state can emerge.

But you no longer need to sit, wait and hope for this state to happen upon you. Nor do you need to follow the Rolling Stones around the world to experience this deep connection with life. It is here for you always. The mind will do its utmost to distract you from this state, because it fears the loss of power and attention it will experience. Still, this state is your natural state. It is what all the mystics and masters have been pointing to ever since humans lost it in thought. Let today be the beginning of your return to this natural, spacious, joyful oneness.

Day 7: Making a Commitment

Time to Wake Up

When we make the commitment to wake up, our belief that happiness is outside us gets turned on its head. We make a shift, determined to look for happiness in the inner world. All wisdom, all knowledge and all understanding are inside already – all we have to do is remember it or rediscover it.

If you make waking up the focus of your life, ironically the everyday things that previously absorbed your attention will be taken care of with skill and ease. You will find yourself more productive at work, more loving in your relationships and happy, no matter what. Nothing needs to change, except the awareness of who you are.

It is important that you verify this against your own experience, lest this remain an idea, a belief, or another concept for the mind to play with. Don't settle for a thought. Go inside and experience this world for yourself.

That's all you need to do. Keep turning your focus inward and using the opportunities life gives you to move inside again and again.

There is nothing complicated about this. It is not spiritual or religious, but sometimes I refer to religion and spirituality because I think they're helpful. They provide some nice quotes and stories that can point us in the right direction. But all we are doing is this: noticing and watching and experiencing.

Why the World Can't Make You Happy (for Long)

Of course, there is no way that the outside world can make you happy. It can give you what you want now and then, but it can't make you happy. It's not meant to. And it doesn't need to, because happiness is in you – happiness is you – it is who you are. The outside world can't give you who you are. You experience who you are when you wake up from 'sinking through thinking'. Then the outside world is a really fun place. It's really enjoyable.

I can say this confidently because I experience both sides regularly. I experience moments of 'Wow, this isn't real. This is just a story, but it sure is fun!' I also experience moments when the story feels real and stressful. I'm in a state of half-sleep, and I feel hungover and lethargic.

But when I wake up and live in that awakeness, the world is so alive and so invigorating that it's incredible. You will laugh when you live in this awakeness. Often, in fact, people who have discovered it say, 'I seem to be laughing a lot more.'

The Un-goal

It is incredibly freeing to make waking up your only goal, or perhaps we should call it an un-goal, as it cannot be achieved in the future. Once you embrace this journey of waking up, worldly troubles become less worrisome, and it doesn't even matter if you fall asleep again for a while.

I have days of getting caught up in thought and emotion, but when I wake up, I don't really care about all that. It was an experience, and it is finished. I will use the experience to continue to wake up and to strengthen my remembering.

The End of Progress

When you know that's all there is to it, you can forget about progress because, in the moment, you're either awake out of thought or you're lost in thought. If you're lost in it, you won't know, because you'll be in the fog of thought. If you are not lost in it, then you are awake, and there is nothing else to do. Just sit in that. You will fall asleep again, and you will wake up again, and fall asleep again, and wake up again.

Activity: No Progress, No Problem

Close your eyes for a moment or two and completely renounce progress. Take a breath and make that breath everything, forget about any future improvement and just sit. Be watchful for future focused thoughts, and when they arise, let them go past untouched, just watch.

Open your eyes and keep breathing mindfully. Let your body sink into the chair and for a moment act as if the universe is your servant and will bring you whatever you need at precisely the right moment. Further, pretend that the universe is such a brilliant servant that you don't even need to think about or ask for what you need, that it instinctively knows exactly what to deliver exactly when, and that no consideration from you is necessary. With this pressure removed, breathe, enjoy and let this moment take care of itself.

Could it be that the present moment is such a servant? That everything you have experienced happened at exactly the right instant because it was exactly what you needed? If you stop arguing with Now for a while, you will find that this is true. We are like a passenger on a commercial flight who sits worrying about how much fuel might be left, what turbulence lies ahead and whether the cabin pressure will hold. This is a stressful way to travel. Much better to make enjoying this moment your focus and let the pilot take you where you need to go.

And so the commitment to waking up is a commitment to let go of everything that is not yours to hold. It is a deep sense of allowing the dance to move as it does, of letting life be the expert and remaining the curious, engaged beginner, always. All we are committing to is to concern ourselves with one question: where is my attention in this instant? The only worthwhile concern is this: are you awake, engaged in this beautiful instant?

Conclusion

And so, we come to the end of our journey together. Or is it the beginning? Over the course of this journey, we have explored some interesting discoveries. We have discovered the root of unhappiness – thinking about the past and the future – and the simple solution – experiencing life this instant. We have learnt the power of allowfulness, and perhaps most importantly, we have learnt that we are who we think we are. Discovering that, in fact, thought is something that happens, not who you are, can be confusing, empowering and joyful.

Now it's up to you. You have the skills to bring peace into this world. You have a series of exercises to use any time you want, and most of all you have awareness, that underlying peace that is who you are. Now that you know this, you can return to it whenever you want, and as you become more intimate with this fact, that peace only deepens.

If you have any questions or struggles on your journey, remember the resources at www.olidoyle.com/MFL. There you can sign up for my newsletter to receive resources and tips, and to keep in touch with your queries along the way. You

can also email me at oli@peacethroughmindfulness.com.au –
I love hearing from readers.

Your happiness depends on nothing outside you. It is your
birthright and your destiny.

May you find peace, and may you bring peace into this
world.

Thank You

Without my amazing wife Ren, this book would be a pale shadow of what it is. Thank you always. Likewise our two crazy kids, Liam and Freya, continuously remind me that the here and now is where I should be.

Thanks to my parents James and Tricia, my brother Phil and my sister Abby for your support and for sharing this experience called life.

My work is inspired by a few people who won't even realise it. I would like to thank Carolyn, Llevellyse, Janet, Jen, Ellen and Julia, your stories keep reminding me of why I do this.

Thanks to Jess, Jaz, Karen, Kris, Kate, Anne, Chris and Sue, for making the daytime fun.

I would like to thank my spiritual teachers, some of you I have met, others I have not. Everlasting thanks go to Ekai Korematsu Osho, Eckhart Tolle, Byron Katie, Osho and Adyashanti. I bow at the feet of Bodhidharma, Mahakashyapa, Gautama Buddha and all who contributed to the meditation traditions of the world. Your gift is truly lasting.

Thank you to Jane Graham Maw for being my guide through this process. And finally, thanks to Jillian Young and the team at Orion for seeing something they wanted to be a part of. I hope that together we can share this work far and wide.

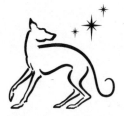